Editor
Paul S. Giacomini

Case Studies in Multiple Sclerosis

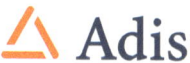

Editor
Professor Paul S. Giacomini
Montreal Neurological Hospital and Institute
McGill University Health Centre
McGill University
Montreal, Quebec, Canada

ISBN 978-3-319-31188-3 ISBN 978-3-319-31190-6 (eBook)
DOI 10.1007/978-3-319-31190-6

Printed on acid-free paper

This Adis imprint is published by Springer Nature
The registered company is Springer International Publishing AG Switzerland

Project editor: Katrina Dorn

Case Studies in Multiple Sclerosis

Acknowledgements

I am very grateful to my many colleagues who have generously contributed to this work by authoring cases, and in doing so, sharing their wisdom, knowledge and experience in the management of patients with multiple sclerosis. I am also grateful to Dr. Jack Antel and Dr. Liam Durcan of McGill University, my friends and mentors of many years, who first kindled my interest in neurology and continue to serve as role models to this day.

This book is dedicated to my family, my wife Valerie and my two children, Katie and Jack, for their unwavering love and support over the years, and for putting up with both my presence and absence alike. I am eternally grateful for their devotion and patience that seem to know no bounds.

Contents

PEDIATRIC MULTIPLE SCLEROSIS AND RELATED DISORDERS

OTHER MULTIPLE SCLEROSIS-RELATED DISORDERS

Author biography

Professor Paul S. Giacomini is a neurologist with expertise in multiple sclerosis and neuro-inflammatory disorders, as well as advanced neuroimaging techniques. He studied medicine at the University of Toronto and returned to his native Montreal to pursue his neurology residency at McGill University, followed by a clinical fellowship in multiple sclerosis, and post-doctoral studies evaluating non-conventional neuroimaging techniques in multiple sclerosis. He is currently a faculty member of McGill University, an Assistant Professor of Neurology and Neurosurgery, and an attending physician at the Montreal Neurological Institute (MNI). He also serves as the Director of the McGill Neurology Fellowship Program in Multiple Sclerosis and Neuro-Inflammatory Disorders, and as the Associate Director of the MNI Multiple Sclerosis Clinic. In addition to an active clinical practice specializing in multiple sclerosis and related disorders, Professor Giacomini has served as a principal investigator in numerous clinical trials evaluating novel therapeutics in relapsing and progressive multiple sclerosis. He is also involved in neuroimmunology translational research aimed at better understanding the mechanism of action of multiple sclerosis therapeutics. He is very active in continuing medical education, lecturing locally and nationally on the management of multiple sclerosis and related disorders.

Contributors

Mahtab Ghadiri, MBBS, FRACP
Montreal Neurological Hospital
and Institute
McGill University
Montreal, Quebec, Canada

Anne-Marie Trudelle, MD,
FRCPC
Montreal Neurological Hospital
and Institute
McGill University
Montreal, Quebec, Canada

Christopher Eckstein, MD
Duke University School
of Medicine
Durham, North Carolina, USA

Scott Newsome, D.O.
Johns Hopkins School
of Medicine
Johns Hopkins Hospital
Baltimore, Maryland, USA

Sarah A. Morrow, MD, MS,
FRCPC
London Health Sciences Multiple
Sclerosis Clinic
University of Western Ontario
London, Ontario, Canada

Sunita Venkateswaran, MD,
FRCPC
Children's Hospital of
Eastern Ontario
University of Ottawa
Ottawa, Ontario, Canada

Matthew R. Lincoln, MD, PhD
University of Toronto
Toronto, Ontario, Canada

Jiwon Oh, MD, PhD, FRCPC
St. Michael's Hospital
Keenan Research Centre
Li Ka Shing Knowledge Institute
University of Toronto
Toronto, Ontario, Canada

Elias S. Sotirchos, MD
Johns Hopkins Hospital
Baltimore, Maryland, USA

Shiv Saidha, MBBCh, MD,
MRCPI
Johns Hopkins Hospital
Baltimore, Maryland, USA

Preface

The treatment of multiple sclerosis (MS) is in the midst of a therapeutic revolution with the emergence of several new therapies over the last decade. This expanding treatment landscape has resulted in more options for patients, but has also increased the complexity of care. The objective of this book is to help neurologists, and neurology residents alike, better appreciate some of the complex issues pertaining to the management of MS, as well as impart some clinical pearls from expert physicians who have faced these same challenges. We have tried to make this book insightful and pragmatic, enabling the reader to better navigate these clinical challenges in their own practice.

Clinically Isolated
Syndrome

Optic neuritis

Mahtab Ghadiri

History

A 27-year-old Caucasian female presented with subacute painful monocular visual loss. Over 4 days, she developed discomfort in the left eye, made worse with eye movements, followed by progressive blurring of left eye vision. There were no right eye symptoms and no previous ocular history. She had been systemically well, with no recent infections or vaccinations. While giving a detailed history, she recalled fleeting episodes of limb paresthesia lasting minutes, with no other history of transient neurological symptoms. She was a smoker with a past history of asthma but took no regular medications. She had a cousin with multiple sclerosis (MS) and was very concerned about her own risk of developing the condition.

Examination

A left relative afferent pupillary defect was noted. Visual acuity was 20/20 on the right eye and 20/40 on the left. Visual fields were full to confrontation. Fundoscopy revealed normal fundi. There was left eye red desaturation and abnormal color vision on Ishihara plate testing. The remainder of the cranial nerve examination was normal. Limb examination revealed mildly brisk (3+) symmetrical deep tendon reflexes and flexor plantar responses. Strength, coordination, and sensation were normal, as was a gait examination. A systemic examination was unremarkable.

© Springer International Publishing Switzerland 2017
P.S. Giacomini (ed.), *Case Studies in Multiple Sclerosis*,
DOI 10.1007/978-3-319-31190-6_1

Investigations

A gadolinium contrast-enhanced MRI of the brain and orbits was obtained (Figure 1.1). Hyperintensity on T2-weighted images and contrast enhancement on the T1-weighted images of the left optic nerve was noted. No cerebral lesions were detected. An MRI of the spine with gadolinium contrast was reported as normal.

A subsequent cerebrospinal fluid (CSF) examination was normal, with no leukocytes or oligoclonal bands detected. Basic biochemistry, complete blood count, B_{12}, folate, and inflammatory markers were all normal. Serum antinuclear antibody and aquaporin-4 antibody tests were also negative.

Outcome

The diagnosis for this patient is left-sided optic neuritis and a clinically isolated syndrome (CIS).

Discussion

The term CIS describes a single episode of neurological symptoms and signs suggestive of an inflammatory demyelinating CNS lesion and, most commonly, is the first presentation of MS. The time course of CIS follows that of a typical MS relapse: acute to subacute onset, reaching a peak

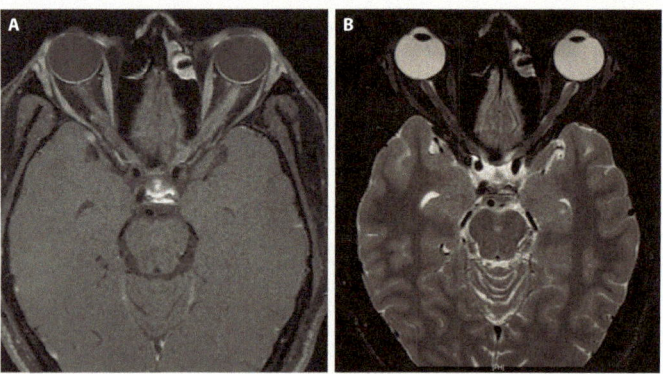

Figure 1.1 Gadolinium-enhanced (A) T1 and (B) T2 MRI showing left optic nerve enhancement and T2 hyperintensity.

from within days to up to 2–3 weeks, followed by a plateau in symptoms, and then a gradual improvement over several weeks. A number of features of this case were suggestive of typical MS. The patient belongs to the most common demographic group for MS presentation: a woman between 20–40 years of age. Her presentation with optic neuritis is also typical, as this is a common presenting feature of MS, as are episodes of myelitis and brainstem syndromes.

Typical features of optic neuritis are unilateral mild ocular pain on eye movement, reduced color vision and visual acuity, a relative afferent pupillary defect, and a normal optic disc (or mild disc swelling). Color vision, easily tested with Ishihara plates, is almost always abnormal in the presence of reduced visual acuity, and is also abnormal in 50% of cases of optic neuritis with normal visual acuity [1]. Unusual features such as bilateral involvement, optic disc hemorrhage, severe pain, painless visual loss, or lack of light perception should raise suspicions for an alternative diagnosis. None of these atypical features were present in this case. In typical optic neuritis, symptoms develop over days and begin to improve within several weeks, with favorable long-term outcomes in the majority of cases [2].

Basic investigations for systemic inflammatory diseases, treatable nutritional deficiencies (especially B_{12} deficiency), and aquaporin-4 antibody for neuromyelitis optica were reasonable tests to rule out alternative diagnoses in this case. In atypical cases, or where additional clues are present on history or examination, a more extensive screen for differential diagnoses such as sarcoidosis, connective tissue diseases, infection, or paraneoplastic disorders may be indicated.

Conversion to multiple sclerosis

Widely accepted MS diagnostic criteria are based on the demonstration of disease dissemination in time and in space. MRI has become integral to the diagnosis of MS and in the most recent revision of the criteria (Table 1.1) a diagnosis of MS can be made at the time of a CIS with the aid of MRI criteria for dissemination in time and space [3]. In this case, however, while radiological evidence of the optic neuritis was seen, no MRI evidence for dissemination of disease in time or space was found.

Clinical presentation	Additional data needed for multiple sclerosis (MS) diagnosis
≥2 attacks; objective clinical evidence of ≥2 lesions or objective clinical evidence of 1 lesion with reasonable historical evidence of a prior attack	None
≥2 attacks; objective clinical evidence of 1 lesion	Dissemination in space (DIS), demonstrated by: • ≥1 T2 lesion in at least 2 of 4 MS-typical regions of the CNS (periventricular, juxtacortical, infratentorial, or spinal cord) *Or* • Await a further clinical attack implicating a different CNS site
1 attack; objective clinical evidence of ≥2 lesions	Dissemination in time (DIT), demonstrated by: • Simultaneous presence of asymptomatic gadolinium-enhancing and nonenhancing lesions at any time *Or* • A new T2 and/or gadolinium-enhancing lesion(s) on follow-up MRI, irrespective of its timing with reference to a baseline scan *Or* • Second clinical attack
1 attack; objective clinical evidence of 1 lesion (monosymptomatic presentation; clinically isolated syndrome)	DIS and DIT, demonstrated by: For DIS: • ≥1 T2 lesion in at least 2 of 4 MS-typical regions of the CNS (periventricular, juxtacortical, infratentorial, or spinal cord) *Or* • Await a second clinical attack implicating a different CNS site *And* For DIT: • Simultaneous presence of asymptomatic gadolinium-enhancing and nonenhancing lesions at any time *Or* • A new T2 and/or gadolinium-enhancing lesion(s) on follow-up MRI, irrespective of its timing with reference to a baseline scan *Or* • Await a second clinical attack
Insidious neurologic progression suggestive of MS (primary progressive MS)	1 year of disease progression (retrospectively or prospectively determined), plus 2 of 3 of the following criteria: • Evidence for DIS in the brain based on ≥1 T2 lesions in the MS-characteristic (periventricular, juxtacortical, or infratentorial) regions • Evidence for DIS in the spinal cord based on ≥2 T2 lesions in the cord • Positive CSF (isoelectric focusing evidence of oligoclonal bands and/or elevated immunoglobulin G index)

Table 1.1 2010 McDonald criteria for the diagnosis of multiple sclerosis. CNS, central nervous system; CSF, cerebrospinal fluid. Reproduced with permission from Polman et al [3] ©Wiley.

Assessment of the risk of relapse and conversion to MS is paramount in cases of CIS as not all patients with a CIS will go on to develop MS. Reported rates of conversion to MS vary widely between studies (10–85%) [4–7]. Patients of younger age and female sex, as in this case, have a higher risk of conversion to MS, as do non-white patients. However, the most powerful tool for prognosticating risk of MS is the MRI, which demonstrates asymptomatic lesions in 50–70% of cases of CIS [8,9]. The long-term risk of conversion to MS increases from around 20% with a normal baseline MRI brain, as found in this case, to 60–80% with an abnormal MRI [4,5,10]. The risk of MS is also higher with a greater number of lesions [11], and with lesions in certain locations, such as infratentorial lesions [6]. CSF oligoclonal bands are present in two-thirds of cases of CIS [12]. Their presence increases the risk of conversion to MS, but has been shown to add little to risk stratification in those with multiple MRI lesions, whose risk of MS can already be estimated to be high [13]. However, the absence of oligoclonal bands in patients with CIS and a normal brain MRI, as in this case, confers a low risk of conversion to MS, and a CSF examination is of great value where there are atypical features or diagnostic uncertainty.

Fifteen-year follow-up data from the Optic Neuritis Treatment Trial (ONTT) indicates a 50% overall risk of conversion to MS after optic neuritis [4]. The presence of one or more demyelinating lesions on brain MRI conferred a conversion risk of 72%, compared to 25% with a normal MRI. Notably, the risk of conversion was highest in the first 5 years after optic neuritis and approached zero in those with a normal baseline MRI who reached 10-year follow-up without developing MS [4]. Thus, if the patient in this case is followed for 5 years without developing MS, it is highly likely that they are amongst those patients with a true monophasic optic neuritis.

At the time of a CIS, there are a number of features that can aid in predicting disease course and future disability from MS. A monosymptomatic, purely afferent CIS, as seen in this case, is a good prognostic feature. A polysymptomatic onset or a presentation involving motor impairment confers a greater risk of future disability from MS. The early course of MS is also informative of future disease outcomes. An incomplete recovery from the initial attack, a short interval to a second attack, and a high early relapse rate are poor prognostic indicators. In patients with optic neuritis followed through the ONTT, 15-year outcomes in those developing MS were generally good, with two-thirds having an Expanded Disability Status Scale score of <3.0 [14].

While many genes have a demonstrated association with MS risk, MS pathogenesis is clearly multifactorial and dependent on the interplay of multiple genetic and environmental factors. True familial history of MS is uncommon (~10% of patients with MS) [15]. The sibling of a patient with MS has a 2.7% risk of developing MS, compared to the general population risk of 0.16% [16]. Thus, for this patient, a family history of MS (a cousin) only minimally increases her lifetime risk of developing MS (0.73%) [16], which can be reassuring to the patient. Smoking, however, is an established environmental MS risk factor, with 75% of smokers vs. 51% of non-smokers converting from CIS to MS in a 3-year follow-up study [17]. Thus, this patient should be counselled accordingly.

Treatment

Intravenous methylprednisolone is the standard of care in any CIS when symptom severity warrants acute treatment. In optic neuritis, treatment is often given if there is pain or significant visual loss, and should be offered in this case. Evidence for the use of steroids comes predominantly from the ONTT, which demonstrated a more rapid clinical improvement with intravenous steroids, although visual outcomes at one year were not altered by treatment [18].

Decisions regarding disease-modifying therapy (DMT) for CIS and early MS can be difficult. Studies have shown that treatment of CIS with DMTs extends the time to next relapse and conversion to MS [19–22], but a benefit in regards to long-term disability has not been demonstrated. While many patients with CIS develop MS, a proportion of patients will not go on to have further relapses and treatment of such patients exposes them to the risks of immunotherapy without benefit. Given the lack of major predictors of MS conversion in this case (abnormal MRI or CSF oligoclonal bands), an appropriate course of action would be careful clinical monitoring and a repeat MRI scan in 3–6 months, looking for evidence of disease dissemination in time and space. Early repeat imaging following CIS is useful, rather than clinical monitoring alone, as clinically silent lesions in MS are up to ten times more frequent than symptomatic lesions [23]. Even in cases of CIS such as this one, with a reassuringly normal MRI brain, infrequent follow up and MRI monitoring is advised, at least for the 5-year period of greatest risk of conversion to MS.

Clinical pearls

- A CIS describes an isolated neurological syndrome suggestive of MS and most commonly manifests as optic neuritis, myelitis, or a brainstem syndrome.
- Typical optic neuritis manifests as subacute, painful, monocular loss of visual acuity with loss of color vision and is usually associated with a good visual recovery.
- When warranted due to symptom severity, acute treatment for a CIS is intravenous steroids, which may hasten neurological recovery.
- A gadolinium-enhanced MRI of both the brain and spinal cord at the time of a CIS is the most powerful tool for stratifying risk of conversion to MS and may allow an immediate diagnosis of MS to be made where dissemination in time and space are demonstrated.
- While a CSF examination is not essential for diagnosis, particularly in typical cases of CIS, it can be useful where there is diagnostic uncertainty and can also aid in prognostication.
- A number of features of CIS are associated with greater long-term disability from MS, including a polysymptomatic presentation, motor impairment, an incomplete recovery, and a short interval from CIS to second attack.
- Close monitoring (eg, repeat MRIs) are indicated following a CIS, as subclinical disease activity is common in MS and often demonstrable radiologically.
- While treatment of CIS with DMTs for MS has been shown to extend the time to relapse and development of MS, a long-term disability benefit has not been demonstrated.

References

1 The clinical profile of optic neuritis. Experience of the Optic Neuritis Treatment Trial. Optic Neuritis Study Group. *Arch Ophthalmol.* 1991;109:1673-1678.

2 Beck RW, Cleary PA, Backlund JC. The course of visual recovery after optic neuritis. Experience of the Optic Neuritis Treatment Trial. *Ophthalmology.* 1994;101:1771-1778.

3 Polman CH, Reingold SC, Banwell B, et al. Diagnostic criteria for multiple sclerosis: 2010 revisions to the McDonald criteria. *Ann Neurol.* 2011;69:292-302.

4 Optic Neuritis Study Group. Multiple sclerosis risk after optic neuritis: final optic neuritis treatment trial follow-up. *Arch Neurol.* 2008;65:727-732.

5 Fisniku LK, Brex PA, Altmann DR, et al. Disability and T2 MRI lesions: a 20-year follow-up of patients with relapse onset of multiple sclerosis. *Brain.* 2008;131:808-817.

6 Tintore M, Rovira A, Arrambide G, et al. Brainstem lesions in clinically isolated syndromes. *Neurology.* 2010;75:1933-1938.

7 Young J, Quinn S, Hurrell M, Taylor B. Clinically isolated acute transverse myelitis: prognostic features and incidence. *Mult Scler.* 2009;15:1295-1302.

8 Jacobs L, Kinkel PR, Kinkel WR. Silent brain lesions in patients with isolated idiopathic optic neuritis. A clinical and nuclear magnetic resonance imaging study. *Arch Neurol.* 1986;43:452-455.

9 Ormerod IE, Bronstein A, Rudge P, et al. Magnetic resonance imaging in clinically isolated lesions of the brain stem. *J Neurol Neurosurg Psychiatry.*1986;49:737-743.

10 Tintoré M, Rovira A, Río J, et al. Baseline MRI predicts future attacks and disability in clinically isolated syndromes. *Neurology.* 2006;67:968-972.

11 Miller DH, Chard DT, Ciccarelli O. Clinically isolated syndromes. *Lancet Neurol.* 2012;11:157-169.

12 Miller D, Barkhof F, Montalban X, Thompson A, Filippi M. Clinically isolated syndromes suggestive of multiple sclerosis, part I: natural history, pathogenesis, diagnosis, and prognosis. *Lancet Neurol.* 2005;4:281-288.

13 Tintoré M, Rovira A, Río J, et al. Do oligoclonal bands add information to MRI in first attacks of multiple sclerosis? *Neurology.* 2008;70:1079-1083.

14 Compston A. *McAlpine's Multiple Sclerosis*, 4th edn. Edinburgh: Churchill Livingstone; 2005.

15 OGorman C, Lin R, Stankovich J, Broadley SA. Modelling genetic susceptibility to multiple sclerosis with family data. *Neuroepidemiology.* 2013;40:1-12.

16 Di Pauli F, Reindl M, Ehling R, et al. Smoking is a risk factor for early conversion to clinically definite multiple sclerosis. *Mult Scler.* 2008;14:1026-1030.

17 The Optic Neuritis Study Group. Multiple sclerosis risk after optic neuritis: final optic neuritis treatment trial follow-up. *Arch Neurol.* 2008;65:727-732.

18 Beck RW, Gal RL. Treatment of acute optic neuritis: a summary of findings from the optic neuritis treatment trial. *Arch Ophthalmol.* 2008;126:994-995.

19 Comi G, Martinelli V, Rodegher M, et al. Effect of glatiramer acetate on conversion to clinically definite multiple sclerosis in patients with clinically isolated syndrome (PreCISe study): a randomised, double-blind, placebo-controlled trial. *Lancet* 1931;374:1503-1511.

20 Kappos L, Polman CH, Freedman MS, et al. Treatment with interferon beta-1b delays conversion to clinically definite and McDonald MS in patients with clinically isolated syndromes. *Neurology.* 2006;67:1242-1249.

21 Comi G, Filippi M, Barkhof F, et al. Effect of early interferon treatment on conversion to definite multiple sclerosis: a randomised study. *Lancet.* 2001;357:1576-1582.

22 Jacobs LD, Beck RW, Simon JH, et al. Intramuscular interferon beta-1A therapy initiated during a first demyelinating event in multiple sclerosis. *N Engl J Med.* 2000;343:898-904.

23 Willoughby EW, Grochowski E, Li DKB, Oger J, Kastrukoff LF, Paty DW. Serial magnetic resonance scanning in multiple sclerosis: A second prospective study in relapsing patients. *Ann Neurol.* 1989;25:43-49.

Myelitis

Mahtab Ghadiri

History

A 42-year-old man presented to the emergency department with altered sensation in the lower limbs and difficulty ambulating. He first noted paresthesia in his feet 1 week prior. The altered sensation gradually ascended to involve the length of both legs and his trunk to around the umbilicus. Over the preceding 2 days, he had noticed some difficulty walking longer distances and climbing stairs and had developed a sensation of incomplete bladder emptying. He had been systemically well and there was no prior history of neurological symptoms. He had a background history of mild hypertension but took no medication. There was no relevant family history.

Examination

Lower limb examination revealed non-sustained ankle clonus bilaterally, with brisk knee jerks and extensor plantar reflexes. There was mild weakness of left hip flexion and ankle dorsiflexion bilaterally. Pinprick sensation was decreased throughout the lower limbs, with a sensory level at approximately T9. There was reduction of distal proprioception and vibration sense. Examination of gait revealed difficulty walking on heels and performing a squat-to-stand manoeuvre. The upper limb and cranial nerve examinations were normal and there were no cerebellar signs. The systemic examination was unremarkable.

© Springer International Publishing Switzerland 2017
P.S. Giacomini (ed.), *Case Studies in Multiple Sclerosis*,
DOI 10.1007/978-3-319-31190-6_2

Investigations

An MRI of the spine (Figure 2.1) revealed a T2 hyperintense cord lesion, extending from T2 to T5, with associated gadolinium enhancement. A brain MRI (Figure 2.2) revealed multiple T2 hyperintense white matter lesions, including callosal lesions, periventricular lesions extending perpendicular to the ventricles consistent with 'Dawson's fingers', and a left cerebellar lesion. Faint gadolinium enhancement of one periventricular lesion was noted.

A cerebrospinal fluid (CSF) examination revealed 47 mononuclear cells/μL and a normal protein level. CSF culture and viral polymerase chain reaction (PCR) analyses were negative, while CSF oligoclonal bands were positive. A blood screen for multiple sclerosis (MS) mimics was performed, including inflammatory markers, vitamin B_{12}, methylmalonic

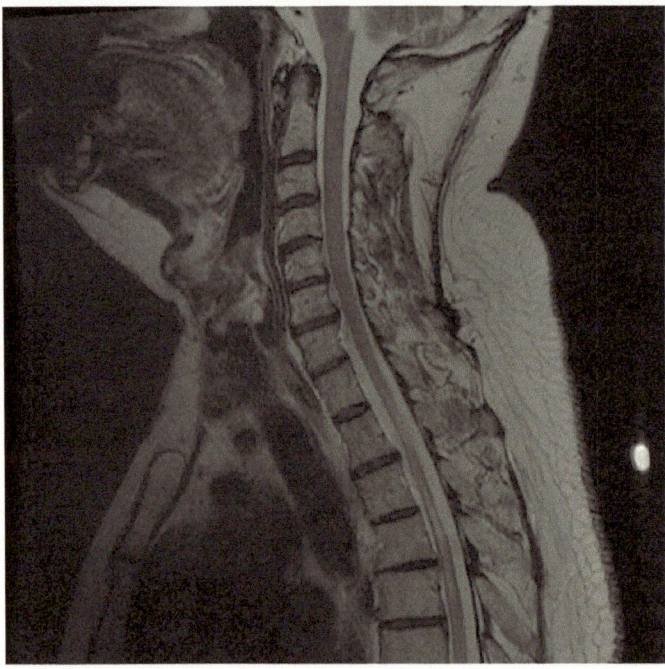

Figure 2.1 An axial T2-weighted MRI of the cervical spinal cord showing a hyperintense lesion extending from T2 to T5.

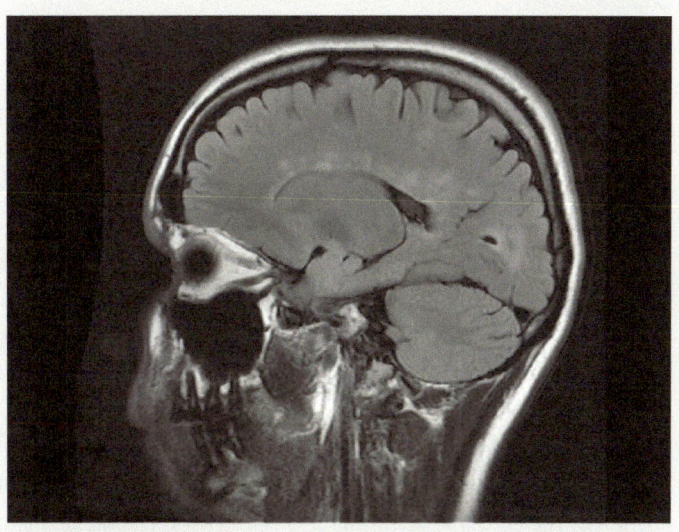

Figure 2.2 A sagittal FLAIR image of the brain showing multiple hyperintense white matter lesions, including 'Dawson's fingers.'

acid, folate, copper studies, aquaporin-4 antibodies, syphilis serology, angiotensin-converting enzyme, antinuclear antibodies, extractable nuclear antibodies, antineutrophil cytoplasmic antibodies, rheumatoid factor, double-stranded DNA antibodies, and antiphospholipid antibodies, all of which were normal or negative.

Outcome

This patient presented with myelitis and, given the absence of previous episodes of neurological symptoms, can be diagnosed with a clinically isolated syndrome (CIS). Following management of this acute episode and discussion of the diagnosis, the patient can be considered for commencement of a disease-modifying therapy (DMT), as there is established evidence for decreased relapse rates, slower accumulation of lesions, and reduced long-term disability with early treatment of MS. Given the presence of some unusual features in this case, reassessment of the diagnosis and repeat evaluation for a potential MS mimic should be considered in the future if his disease course or treatment response is atypical.

Discussion

The presence of brain lesions typical for MS strengthens the likelihood of underlying MS, although other diseases can mimic MS, both clinically and radiologically. In cases of CIS with features typical for MS, minimal testing may be required to help exclude alternative diagnoses, such as blood tests for inflammatory markers, antinuclear antibodies, and a nutritional deficiency screen (eg, Vitamin B_{12}, folate). While more extensive screening for MS mimics is not warranted in all cases of CIS, when atypical features are present, as in this case, a thorough search for differential diagnoses is warranted. Distinguishing a first presentation of MS from other mimics is important, as the use of MS therapies in other disorders can be both ineffective and even potentially harmful.

Typical myelitis related to MS is partial, usually affecting a peripheral portion of the cord and spanning less than two vertebral segments on imaging, and resulting in incomplete and often asymmetrical symptoms and signs below the level of the lesion. As with symptomatic lesions in other areas, symptoms and signs of MS myelitis tend to progress over days to several weeks, typically with ascending sensory changes, sphincter dysfunction, and mild-to-moderate lower limb weakness. Severe weakness, complete myelitis, and cauda equina syndrome are unusual in MS. Patients with acute partial myelitis are at an increased risk of recurrence and transition to MS [1]. On the other hand, complete myelitis, affecting all ascending and descending spinal tracts and usually resulting from a full-thickness lesion of the spinal cord, is uncommon in MS.

The differential diagnosis for myelitis is broad and includes infections, parainfectious myelitis, paraneoplastic syndromes, drug/toxin-induced myelitis, neurosarcoidosis, myelitis associated with systemic autoimmune diseases, and other inflammatory central nervous system diseases, including neuromyelitis optica (NMO) and acute disseminated encephalomyelitis. In 15–30% of cases of myelitis, no underlying cause can be determined [2].

In this case, the patient does not fit the stereotypical demographics for a new diagnosis of MS, being male and older than the usual age of onset of MS (20–40 years) [1]. The CSF pleocytosis is unusual; the cell count is often normal and very rarely greater than 50 cells/μL in MS. While oligoclonal bands are present in up to 95% of cases of MS [3], they are not wholly specific for MS and may be seen in other inflammatory and infectious diseases.

The presence of a longitudinally extensive cord lesion (LETM), or a cord lesion spanning more than three vertebral segments on imaging, is also unusual in MS. On axial sections, LETM usually involves the central cord, unlike the typical eccentric lesions seen in MS, and may produce greater cord swelling than MS cord lesions. A number of diagnoses should be considered in the setting of LETM, although the most important of these are the NMO spectrum disorders. The aquaporin-4 antibody test, negative in this case, is positive in up to 89% of NMO cases [4]. Other clues to NMO are also absent in this patient, such as evidence of optic neuritis or distinctive brain MRI features, such as periependymal or area postrema lesions. Other causes of LETM, such as neurosarcoidosis, parainfectious and connective tissue diseases also appear unlikely given the lack of supportive features on history, examination, or blood tests.

Importantly, the MRI in this case fulfills the McDonald criteria (see Table 1.1) for both dissemination in time (DIT) and dissemination in space (DIS). Acute lesions in MS may show gadolinium enhancement for several weeks, thus the presence of both asymptomatic enhancing and nonenhancing lesions on a single MRI demonstrates lesions of differing chronicity and establishes DIT. MRI criteria for DIS require the presence of lesions in at least two of four regions typically affected in MS; in this case, three of the regions are involved radiologically (periventricular, infratentorial, and spinal cord). The McDonald criteria for MS also require that there is no better explanation for a patient's presentation, as the MRI criteria alone can be fulfilled by other disorders [5]. As the search for alternative diagnoses has been negative and the brain MRI lesions and CSF findings are suggestive, the most likely cause of this patient's CIS is MS.

Whilst initially difficult, receiving an earlier diagnosis of MS reduces patient anxiety related to diagnostic uncertainty and is preferred by patients, according to survey results [6,7].

Clinical pearls

- Spinal cord involvement in MS usually manifests as a partial myelitis, with incomplete and often asymmetrical involvement of ascending and descending tracts.

- Typical MS brain lesions are small ovoid T2 hyperintense lesions of the deep white matter, corpus callosum, and periventricular (including 'Dawson's fingers'), juxtacortical, and infratentorial regions. Spinal cord lesions in MS are typically short-segment lesions of the peripheral part of the cord.

- A thorough search for MS mimics is warranted in cases of CIS when there are atypical clinical or radiological features. The investigative approach must be tailored to the clinical presentation, but may include tests targeting vascular, inflammatory, connective tissue, infective, paraneoplastic, metabolic, and granulomatous diseases.

- Cases of CIS are by definition isolated in time. However, the presence of both asymptomatic nonenhancing and enhancing lesions on a single MRI is sufficient to fulfil DIT criteria for MS. DIS can be demonstrated by MRI lesions in more than one of four regions commonly affected in MS.

- An early diagnosis of MS allows consideration of early commencement of a DMT, which has been associated with a reduction in relapses and decreased long-term disability.

References

1   Beh SC, Greenberg BM, Frohman T, Frohman EM. Transverse myelitis. [Review]. *Neurol Clin.* 2013;31:79-138.

2   de Seze J, Stojkovic T, Breteau G, et al. Acute myelopathies. *Brain.* 2001 1;124:1509-1521.

3   Dobson R, Ramagopalan S, Davis A, Giovannoni G. Cerebrospinal fluid oligoclonal bands in multiple sclerosis and clinically isolated syndromes: a meta-analysis of prevalence, prognosis and effect of latitude. *J Neurol Neurosurg Psychiatry.* 2013;84:909-914.

4   Jiao Y, Fryer JP, Lennon VA, et al. Cerebrospinal fluid oligoclonal bands in multiple sclerosis and clinically isolated syndromes: a meta-analysis of prevalence, prognosis and effect of latitude serostatus and outcome in recurrent longitudinally extensive transverse myelitis. *JAMA Neurol.* 2014;71:48-54.

5   Polman CH, Reingold SC, Banwell B, et al. Diagnostic criteria for multiple sclerosis: 2010 revisions to the McDonald criteria. *Ann Neurol.* 2011;69:292-302.

6   Mushlin AI, Mooney C, Grow V, Phelps CE. The value of diagnostic information to patients with suspected multiple sclerosis. Rochester-Toronto MRI Study Group. *Arch Neurol.* 1994;51:67-72.

7   Heesen C, Kolbeck J, Gold SM, Schulz H, Schulz KH. Delivering the diagnosis of MS -- results of a survey among patients and neurologists. *Acta Neurologica Scand.* 2003;107:363-368.

Early Multiple Sclerosis

Disease-modifying therapies

Anne-Marie Trudelle

History

A 25-year-old man was evaluated in the neurology outpatient clinic for evaluation of a new diagnosis of relapsing-remitting multiple sclerosis (RRMS). He was previously well, not taking any medications, and had no allergies. He described a first episode of right optic neuritis 2 years prior that was treated with intravenous methylprednisolone and from which he recovered completely. Three months ago he had a second episode of cervical transverse myelitis that had improved but did not fully resolve. He noted residual weakness and stiffness in his legs at the time of his evaluation.

Examination

Upon neurological examination he was found to have a right relative afferent pupillary defect, brisk reflexes in all four limbs, upgoing plantar reflexes bilaterally, mild proximal weakness, and moderate spasticity in both lower limbs. Tone and power were normal in the upper extremities. The remaining neurological and physical examination was normal.

Investigations

The patient had a brain MRI that revealed multiple hyperintense lesions on T2-weighted imaging in typical locations for a demyelinating disease. The lesions were located in the periventricular white matter of both cerebral

© Springer International Publishing Switzerland 2017
P.S. Giacomini (ed.), *Case Studies in Multiple Sclerosis*,
DOI 10.1007/978-3-319-31190-6_3

hemispheres, along the corpus callosum, and in the right cerebellar hemisphere. There were no enhancing lesions after gadolinium injection.

The patient had a cervical and thoracic spine MRI that revealed a hyperintense T2 lesion in the cervical spinal cord at the level of C4. There was no swelling or enhancement following gadolinium injection.

The patient had visual evoked potentials that revealed an increased P100 latency on the right side that was compatible with a right anterior visual pathway lesion.

Outcome

Given his young age and the fact he is accumulating neurological disability with each relapse, this patient was offered a disease-modifying therapy (DMT) by his treating physician. It is common practice to advocate for early intervention with a DMT as this provides the best opportunity to reduce relapse-associated disability and potentially leads to less long-term disability.

Discussion

DMTs should be offered to all patients diagnosed with RRMS. The aim of DMT treatment is to decrease the risk of relapses, as well as the accrual of new lesions on MRI, with the overall goal of slowing disability progression [1]. Recently, the concept of 'no evidence of disease activity' (NEDA) has become increasingly adopted as a therapeutic target for all patients initiating DMT treatment for RRMS, as well as an outcome measure in more recent clinical trials [2]. NEDA is defined by three elements: no evidence of relapses, no sustained progression of disability, and no new lesions on an MRI [2]. Early initiation of therapies increases the likelihood of achieving NEDA, but close clinical and radiological vigilence is warranted to monitor treatment response [2].

To date, there are ten approved DMTs for RRMS. Selecting which DMT is right for which patient is a highly individualized process. All medications have their own efficacy, risks, and side-effect profiles, and these characteristics need to be taken into account when discussing options with patients. Compliance is critical to success and thus patient engagement and involvement in the selection process is generally helpful. Numerous factors, including the efficacy of

Medication	Dose	Mechanisms of action	Clinical efficacy	Side effects (most common)	Adverse events
Alemtuzumab (Lemtrada®)[1-3]	12 mg IV daily for 5 days; 12 mg IV daily for 3 days 12 months later	Anti-CD52 monoclonal antibody	Comparison to interferon beta-1a SC: 1. ARR: • 74% reduction[1] • 55% reduction[2] • 49% reduction[3] 2. Confirmed disability progression: • 71% reduction[1] • 42% reduction[3]	Infusion-associated reactions: • headache • rash • fever • urticaria • flushing • nausea • chills	Serious infusion reactions: • cardiac arrythmias • hypotension • hypertension Infections Cytopenias Secondary autoimmunity (thyroid disorders, ITP, nephropathies)
Dimethyl fumarate (Tecfidera®)[4]	240 mg po twice daily	Presumed activation of the Nrf2 transcriptional pathway	Compared to placebo : 1. ARR: • 53% reduction 2. Confirmed disability progression at 2 years: • 38% reduction	Flushing Diarrhea Nausea Abdominal pain Vomiting Pruritus Rash	Lymphopenia PML Proteinuria Elevation in liver enzymes

Table 3.1 Disease-modifying therapies in relapsing-remitting multiple sclerosis (continues overleaf). Disclaimer: this table provides an overview, but is not exhaustive in detail and the medication monographs and source articles should be reviewed thoroughly before making treatment decisions.

Medication	Dose	Mechanisms of action	Clinical efficacy	Side effects (most common)	Adverse events
Fingolimod (Gilenya®)[5]	0.5 mg po daily	Sphingosine-1-phosphate receptor modulator	Compared to placebo: 1. ARR • 54% reduction	Headaches Diarrhea	Infections Lymphopenia Bradyarrhythmia Macular edema Hypertension Elevation of liver enzymes Increased lipids levels Impairment in respiratory function tests PML
Interferon beta-1a (Avonex®, Rebif®)[6,7]	Avonex: • 30 µg IM for 1 week Rebif: • 44 µg SC 3 times per week	Modulates immune response away from pro-inflammatory profile via numerous mechanisms	Compared to placebo: 1. Avonex: • Frequency of exacerbations: – 37% reduction • Time to onset of sustained progression in disability: – 32% reduction 2. Rebif: • Relapse rate: – 52% reduction • Time to onset of progression in disability: – 56% for Rebif compared to 46% for placebo	Flu-like syndrome Injection site cutaneous reactions	Depression Decreased peripheral blood counts Elevation of liver enzymes Thyroid dysfunction Rebif: • TTP-HUS (rare)

Table 3.1 Disease-modifying therapies in relapsing-remitting multiple sclerosis (continues on next page). Disclaimer: this table provides an overview, but is not exhaustive in detail and the medication monographs and source articles should be reviewed thoroughly before making treatment decisions.

Medication	Dose	Mechanisms of action	Clinical efficacy	Side effects (most common)	Adverse events
Interferon beta-1b (Betaseron®)[8,9]	8 MIU SC every other day	Modulates immune response away from pro-inflammatory profile via numerous mechanisms	Compared to placebo: 1. ARR: • 31% reduction	Same as interferon beta-1a	Same as interferon beta-1a
Glatiramer acetate (Copaxone®)[10]	20 mg SC daily	Modulates immune response away from pro-inflammatory profile via numerous mechanisms	Compared to placebo: 1. Relapse-free patients: • 56% compared to 28% in the placebo group 2. Progression-free patients: • 80% compared to 52% in the placebo group	Rare immediate post-injection reaction: • flushing • chest pain • palpitations • anxiety • dyspnea • urticaria Injection site cutaneous reactions	Lipoatrophy Skin necrosis

Table 3.1 Disease-modifying therapies in relapsing-remitting multiple sclerosis (continues overleaf). Disclaimer: this table provides an overview, but is not exhaustive in detail and the medication monographs and source articles should be reviewed thoroughly before making treatment decisions

Medication	Dose	Mechanisms of action	Clinical efficacy	Side effects (most common)	Adverse events
Natalizumab (Tysabri®)[11]	300 mg IV for 4 weeks	Monoclonal antibody; selective adhesion molecule inhibitor (blocks α4-integrin)	Compared to placebo: 1. ARR: • 68% reduction 2. Disability progression: • 54% reduction	Hypersensitivity reactions Infusion reactions: • headache • fatigue • arthralgia • rash • abdominal discomfort	PML Increased liver enzymes Infection
Teriflunomide (Aubagio®)[12,13]	14 mg po daily	Reversible inhibition of the enzyme dihydroorotate dehydrogenase, which is required for the de novo pyrimidine synthesis[12]	Compared to placebo : 1. ARR : • 31.5% RRR[12] • 36.3% RRR[13] 2. Disability progression: • 30% RRR[12] • 31% RRR[13]	Alopecia Diarrhea Nausea	Hypertension Leukopenia Increased liver enzymes Peripheral neuropathy

Table 3.1 Disease-modifying therapies in relapsing-remitting multiple sclerosis (continued). ARR, annualized relapse rate; Gd, gadolinium; IM, intramuscular; ITP, idiopathic thrombocytopenic purpura; IV, intravenously; PML, progressive multifocal leukoencephalopathy; po, taken orally; RR, relative reduction; RRR, relative risk reduction; SC, subcutaneous; TTP-HUS, thrombotic thrombocytic purpura-hemolytic uremic syndrome. Disclaimer: this table provides an overview, but is not exhaustive in detail and the medication monographs and source articles should be reviewed thoroughly before making treatment decisions. See [3-13] for further details regarding the core clinical trials for each medication, including the frequencies of side effects and adverse events.

the therapy, its short- and long-term safety and tolerability profile, patient's medical history and preferences, and disease severity should all influence the choice of a DMT. Table 3.1 summarizes the main available therapies [3–13].

Treatment response with DMTs also needs to be closely monitored. According to the recommendations of one expert panel, the main methods of evaluating treatment response are relapses, disease progression, and MRI activity [1]. The number of relapses occurring on therapy, their severity, and the extent of recovery from the relapses should be assessed. Disease progression can be assessed with the Expanded Disability Status Score (EDSS) and the Timed 25-Foot Walk (T25-FW) [1]. The MRI activity should also be evaluated by determining the number of new gadolinium-enhancing lesions and/or the new T2 lesions per year [1]. Adherence to therapy should also be assessed when monitoring treatment efficacy.

Clinical pearls

- DMTs should be offered to all patients when they are newly diagnosed with RRMS.
- DMTs approved for the treatment of RRMS decrease the number and severity of relapses and decrease the accumulation of new lesions on the MRI, thereby potentially reducing disability progression over time.
- The selection of a specific DMT for a patient is a highly individualized process and takes into account disease severity, patient's history and preferences, efficacy, side-effect profile, and potential long-term treatment complications.
- The monitoring of treatment efficacy can be assessed by measuring relapses (number, severity, and recovery), disease progression (EDSS, T25-FW, clinical progression) and MRI activity (new gadolinium-enhancing lesions or accumulation of new T2 lesions per year).
- Adherence to therapy needs to be addressed when assessing the efficacy of a DMT.

References

1 Freedman MS, Selchen D, Arnold DL, et al; Canadian Multiple Sclerosis Working Group. Treatment optimization in MS: Canadian MS Working Group updated recommendations. *Can J Neurol Sci*. 2013;40:307-323.

2 Imitola J, Racke MK. Is no evidence of disease activity a realistic goal for patients with multiple sclerosis ? *JAMA Neurol*. 2015;72:145-147.

3 Coles AJ, Compston DA, Selmaj KW, et al; CAMMS223 Trial Investigators. Alemtuzumab vs. interferon beta-1a in early multiple sclerosis. *N Engl J Med*. 2008;359:1786-1801.

4 Cohen JA, Coles A, Arnold DL, et al; CARE-MS I investigators. Alemtuzumab versus interferon beta 1a as first-line treatment for patients with relapsing-remitting multiple sclerosis: a randomised controlled phase 3 trial. *Lancet*. 2012;380:1819-1828.

5 Coles AJ, Twyman CL, Arnold DL, et al; CARE-MS II investigators. Alemtuzumab for patients with relapsing multiple sclerosis after disease-modifying therapy: a randomised controlled phase 3 trial. *Lancet*. 2012;380:1829-1839.

6 Gold R, Kappos L, Arnold DL, et al; DEFINE study investigators. Placebo-controlled Phase 3 study of oral BG-12 for relapsing multiple sclerosis. *N Engl J Med*. 2012;367:1098-1107.

7 Kappos L, Radue EW, O'Connor P, et al; FREEDOMS study group. A placebo-controlled trial of oral fingolimod in relapsing multiple sclerosis. *N Engl J Med*. 2010; 362:387-401.

8 Jacobs LD, Cookfair DL, Rudick RA, et al. Intramuscular interferon beta-1a for disease progression in relapsing multiple sclerosis. The Multiple Sclerosis Collaborative Research Group (MSCRG). *Ann Neurol*. 1996;39:285-294.

9 PRISMS Study Group. Randomised double-blind placebo-controlled study of interferon beta-1a in relapsing/remitting multiple sclerosis. PRISMS (Prevention of Relapses and Disability by Interferon beta-1a Subcutaneously in Multiple Sclerosis) Study Group. *Lancet*. 1998;352:1498-1504.

10 Interferon beta-1b is effective in relapsing-remitting multiple sclerosis. I. Clinical results of a multicenter, randomized, double-blind, placebo-controlled trial. The IFNB Multiple Sclerosis Study Group. *Neurology*. 1993;43:655-661.

11 Paty DW, Li DK. Interferon beta-1b is effective in relapsing-remitting multiple sclerosis. MRI analysis results of a multicenter, randomized, double-blind, placebo-controlled trial. UBC MS/ MRI Study Group and the IFNB Multiple Sclerosis Study Group. *Neurology*. 1993;43:662-667.

12 Bornstein MB, Miller A, Slagle S, et al. A pilot trial of cop-1 in exacerbating-remitting multiple sclerosis. *N Engl J Med*. 1987;317:408-414.

13 Polman CH, O'Connor P, Havrdova E, et al. A randomized, placebo-controlled trial of natalizumab for relapsing multiple sclerosis. *N Engl J Med*. 2006;354:899-910.

Management of relapses with corticosteroids

Anne-Marie Trudelle

History

A 28-year-old woman with known relapsing-remitting multiple sclerosis (RRMS) for 2 years was seen in the emergency room for a subacute onset of right-hemibody paresthesia and weakness. Her symptoms had started 3 days prior and were gradually worsening. She was taking an injectable disease-modifying therapy (DMT), glatiramer acetate, that was well tolerated. Her most recent brain MRI was a year ago and her lesion load was stable. She was otherwise in good general health and did not have any infectious symptoms or fever in the weeks preceding her clinical presentation. She had no systemic symptoms and had never experienced these symptoms before.

Examination

The neurological examination performed in the emergency department revealed decreased sensation to pinprick and light touch over the right hemibody. She also felt a 'tingling' sensation, most noticeably over her right hand and foot. She also had moderate limb weakness on her right side. She had brisk (3+) reflexes in her right arm and leg, and left-sided reflexes were normal. The right plantar response was upgoing. She had difficulty walking without assistance and had a clear hemiparetic gait. The remaining neurological examination was intact.

© Springer International Publishing Switzerland 2017
P.S. Giacomini (ed.), *Case Studies in Multiple Sclerosis*,
DOI 10.1007/978-3-319-31190-6_4

Investigations

Blood tests and a urine culture were obtained in the emergency department. The results showed no signs of an acute infection. She underwent
a brain MRI that showed the presence of more than ten hyperintense
T2-weighted imaging lesions that were all compatible with demyelination.
There was one lesion in the cerebellum, one in the medulla, two in the
corpus callosum, and the others were located in the periventricular white
matter of both cerebral hemispheres. In comparison to her previous MRI,
there was one new lesion located in the left corona radiata that was identified following injection of intravenous (IV) gadolinium.

Outcome

This patient is experiencing a multiple sclerosis (MS) relapse. Her clinical
presentation is quite typical, with new neurological deficits evolving
over days; her MRI even shows a new gadolinium-enhancing inflammatory demyelinating lesion, localizing to an area that accounts for
her symptoms. There is no evidence of an intercurrent infection and
she was offered corticiosteroid treatment to help expedite her recovery
from this active relapse.

Discussion

Clinical relapses are the result of focal inflammation and demyelination
in the central nervous sytem, with most showing some degree of subsequent recovery and remyelination [1]. According to the 2010 version of the
McDonald criteria for the diagnosis of MS, a relapse is a "patient-reported
or objectively observed event typical of an acute inflammatory demyelinating event in the central nervous system, current or historical, with
a duration of at least 24 hours, in the absence of fever or infection" [2].
Therefore, the diagnosis of a relapse is largely a clinical diagnosis. The
symptoms will vary depending on the location of the active lesions
within the central nervous system. Common symptoms include sensory
complaints, visual loss (eg, optic neuritis), and weakness. The symptoms
commonly evolve over hours or days and reach a plateau within weeks.
However, symptoms should persist for a minimum of 24 hours in order
to confirm that they are due to a relapse. Recovery usually occurs within

the first 2 or 3 months but patients can still improve up to 12 months after a relapse [3,4].

However, one-third to one-half of all relapses will lead to residual deficits [5]. Residual deficits are most likely to occur if the patient is older than 30 years of age, has a severe relapse with multifocal deficits, and if there is a slow recovery in the first few months following the relapse [6–8]. The average relapse rate for an individual patient is one relapse every 2 years [9]. To help distinguish relapses occurring close to each other, a minimum of 30 days of improvement or stability should separate two relapses [10]. Systemic infection, stressful life events, hormonal fertility treatment, and the postpartum period may increase the risk of relapse [11].

Relapses must be distinguished from paroxysmal symptoms, pseudo-relapses, and daily fluctuations [12]. Paroxysmal symptoms such as trigeminal neuralgia and tonic spasms are usually intermittent and need to occur with increasing frequency or intensity for more than 24 hours to be considered as a relapse [12]. A 'pseudo-relapse' or 'pseudo-exacerbation' is an exacerbation of symptoms from a previous relapse that is occurring in the context of a physiologic stress, such as an increase in body temperature (heat, fever, exercise) or a systemic infection [12]. In these instances, treating the underlying stress, such as the infection, leads to the resolution of the pseudo-relapse symptoms.

The main treatment for relapses in RRMS is the administration of corticosteroids. Corticosteroids act in RRMS by reducing the adhesion molecule production, pro-inflammatory cytokine levels, and circulating CD4 T and B lymphocytes, as well as altering the blood–brain barrier [13,14].

Corticosteroids can be administered either orally or intravenously. A 2012 Cochrane review concluded that there are no significant differences in clinical (benefits and adverse events), radiological, or pharmacological outcomes between intravenous and oral corticosteroids for the treatment of MS relapses [15]. A more recent study showed that oral administration of methylprednisolone 1000 mg daily for 3 days for the treatment of MS relapses was noninferior to IV administration for the improvement of disability scores a month after treatment [16]. Therefore, the route of corticosteroid administration can be decided based on the patient's preference. The dose is usually high, varying between 625–1250 mg daily of oral prednisone or 1000 mg daily of IV methylprednisolone [16–18]. The duration of treatment will vary depending on the route of administration and the dose administered but usually is 3 or 5 days [16–18].

Treatment with corticosteroids in RRMS is generally safe, but systemic infections must be excluded before treatment. Common side effects observed with corticosteroids are weight gain, edema, insomnia, mood disturbances (eg, depression, psychosis), hypertension, impaired glucose tolerance, gastrointestinal upset, pancreatitis, avascular necrosis, myopathy, cataracts, and osteoporosis. Most of these side effects are more common with long-term corticosteroid treatment and are, therefore, probably less common when given in a pulse fashion, as in the treatment of MS relapses. The most common side effects of corticosteroids use for the treatment of MS relapses are insomnia, mood disturbances, and gastrointestinal upset [13].

Severe relapses can be resistant to high-dose oral or intravenous corticosteroids. Some small studies have shown that plasmapheresis is effective and should be considered in the treatment of corticosteroid-resistant MS relapses (level C recommendation by the American Academy of Neurology) [19]. Plasmapheresis can also be offered as an adjunctive treatment of exacerbations in relapsing forms of MS (level B recommendation by the American Academy of Neurology) [19]. Intravenous immunoglobulin (IVIg) can also be considered to treat relapses when steroids are contraindicated and plasmapheresis is not accessible, but the efficacy of IVIg in the treatment of MS relapse is only based on one small study of 17 patients [20]. Therefore, the efficacy of IVIg in treating MS relapses is still unknown [21].

The use of corticosteroids in MS relapses tends to decrease the duration of a relapse but does not seem to alter the long-term outcome of the relapse or the long-term disability from the disease [22]. Corticosteroids were evaluated against placebo in the treatment of MS relapses and there was a significant reduction in short-term disability (based on the Expanded Disability Status Scale Score), along with a 60% increase in the probability of recovery within the first 5 weeks of treatment with corticosteroids [22].

Recognizing relapses is essential because it may help ascertain a diagnosis, enabling the start of DMTs or indicating the need to escalate therapy. It may also be a sign of non-adherence to therapy by the patient.

Clinical pearls

- An MS relapse is defined as a clinical event of symptoms typical of an inflammatory demyelinating episode in the central nervous system that has a duration of at least 24 hours, in the absence of fever or infection.
- The symptoms of an MS relapse will vary depending on where the acute lesions are localized within the central nervous system.
- The main treatment of MS relapses are corticosteroids. They can be administered orally or intravenously. The dose and the duration of the treatment will vary depending on the route of administration.
- Severe MS relapses can be refractory to high-dose corticosteroids. In such cases, plasmapheresis could be considered to treat the MS relapse.
- There are insufficient data to conclude on the efficacy of IVIg in the treatment of MS relapses.
- The treatment of MS relapses with corticosteroids decreases the duration of MS relapses but does not affect long-term disability.
- Recognizing MS relapses is essential to assess the patient's response to treatment, and if escalation of treatment is warranted.

References

1   Noseworthy JH, Lucchinetti C, Rodriguez M, Weinshenker BG. Multiple sclerosis. *New Engl J Med*. 2000;343:938-952.
2   Polman CH, Reingold SC, Banwell B, et al. Diagnostic criteria for multiple sclerosis: 2010 revisions to the McDonald criteria. *Ann Neurol*. 2011; 269:292-302.
3   Hirst CL, Ingram G, Pickersgill TP, et al. Temporal evolution of remission following multiple sclerosis relapse and predictors of outcome. *Mult Scler*. 2012;18:1152-1158.
4   Iuliano G, Napoletano R, Esposito A. Multiple sclerosis: relapses and timing of remissions. *Eur Neurol*. 2008;59:44-48.
5   Lublin FD, Baier M, Cutter G. Effect of relapses on development of residual deficit in multiple sclerosis. *Neurology*. 2003;61:1528-1532.
6   Mowry EM, Pesic M, Grimes B, et al. Demyelinating events in early multiple sclerosis have inherent severity and recovery. *Neurology*. 2009;72:602-608.
7   Vercellino M, Romagnolo A, Mattioda A, et al. Multiple sclerosis relapses: a multivariable analysis of residual disability determinants. *Acta Neurol Scand*. 2009;119:126-130.

8   Leone MA, Bonissoni S, Collimedaglia L, et al. Factors predicting incomplete recovery from relapses in multiple sclerosis: a prospective study. *Mult Scler.* 2008;14:485-493.

9   Confavreux C, Vukusic S. The natural history of multiple sclerosis. *Revue du Practicien.* 2006;56:1313-1320.

10   McDonald WI, Compston A, Edan G, et al. Recommended diagnostic criteria for multiple sclerosis: guidelines from the International Panel on the Diagnosis of Multiple Sclerosis. *Ann Neurol.* 2001;50:121-127.

11   D'hooghe MB, Nagels G, Bissay V, De Keyser J. Modifiable factors influencing relapses and disability in multiple sclerosis. *Mult Scler.* 2010;16:773-785.

12   Galea I, Heesen C. Relapse in multiple sclerosis. *BMJ.* 2015;350:h1765.

13   Andersson P-B, Goodkin DE. Glucocorticosteroid therapy for multiple sclerosis: a critical review. *J Neurol Sci.* 1998;160:16-25.

14   Schweingruber A, Reichardt SD, Reichardt HM. Mechanisms of glucocorticoids in control of neuroinflammation. *J Neuroendocrinol.* 2011;24:174182.

15   Burton JM, O'Connor PW, Hohol M, Beyene J. Oral versus intravenous steroids for treatment of relapses in multiple sclerosis. *Cochrane Database Syst Rev.* 2012;12:CD006921.

16   Le Page E, Veillard D, Laplaud DA, et al. Oral versus intravenous high-dose methylprednisolone for treatment of relapses in patients with multiple sclerosis (COPOUSEP): a randomised, controlled, double-blind, non-inferiority trial. *Lancet.* 2015;386:974-981.

17   Kupersmith MJ, Kaufman D, Paty DW, et al. Megadose corticosteroids in multiple sclerosis. *Neurology.* 1994;44:1.

18   Murray TJ. Diagnosis and treatment of multiple sclerosis. *BMJ.* 2006; 332:525.

19   Cortese I, Chaudhry V, So YT, et al. Evidence-based guideline update: plasmapheresis in neurologic disorders: Report of the Therapeutics and Technology Assessment Subcommittee of the American Academy of Neurology. *Neurology.* 2011;76;294-300.

20   Elovaara I, Kuusisto H, Wu X, et al. Intravenous immunoglobulins are a therapeutic option in the treatment of multiple sclerosis relapse. *Clin Neuropharmacol.* 2011;34:84-89.

21   Goodin DS, Frohman EM, Garmany GP Jr, et al. Disease-modifying therapies in multiple sclerosis: subcommittee of the American Academy of Neurology and the MS Council for Clinical Practice Guidelines. Report of the Therapeutics and Technology Assessment Subcommittee of the American Academy of Neurology and the MS Council for Clinical Practice Guidelines. *Neurology.* 2002;58:169-178.

22   Citterio A, La Mantia L, Ciucci G, Candelise L, Brusaferri F, Midgard R, Filippini G. Corticosteroids or ACTH for acute exacerbations in multiple sclerosis. *Cochrane Database System Rev.* 2000;4:CD001331.

Established Relapsing-Remitting
Multiple Sclerosis

Breakthrough disease

Chris Eckstein

History

A 23-year-old female presented to the clinic for routine follow-up for relapsing remitting multiple sclerosis (RRMS). She was originally diagnosed 2 years prior after a one-month episode of left hand numbness, followed by acute optic neuritis in the right eye, which left her with a significant residual visual acuity deficit despite acute treatment with high-dose intravenous steroids. At that time, a brain MRI revealed multiple nonenhancing white matter lesions in a periventricular pattern consistent with demyelinating disease (Figure 5.1). A lumbar puncture at that time demonstrated oligoclonal bands and mildly elevated cerebrospinal fluid (CSF) protein.

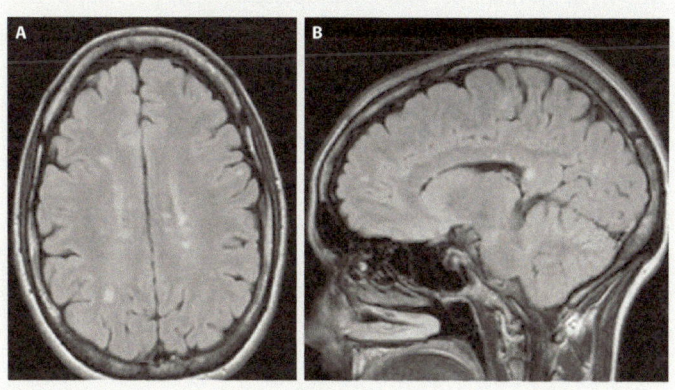

Figure 5.1 Brain MRI in a patient with acute optic neuritis. (A) Axial and **(B)** sagittal FLAIR sequence of the patient's initial MRI demonstrating multiple periventricular white matter lesions consistent with demyelinating disease.

© Springer International Publishing Switzerland 2017
P.S. Giacomini (ed.), *Case Studies in Multiple Sclerosis*,
DOI 10.1007/978-3-319-31190-6_5

She was then started on weekly intramuscular interferon therapy with no further relapses or new brain lesions on her MRI until the current visit.

At this follow-up visit, she reported worsening fatigue and increased blurring of vision in the right eye for about a month. She also noted new gait instability and bilateral leg spasms over the preceding 2–3 weeks. This was relatively mild and did not interfere with her ability to work or complete activities of daily living, but she had never experienced this symptom before. However, she was not overly concerned and attributed her symptoms to a new exercise regimen. The patient denied any fever, chills, night sweats, or dysuria. She had not missed any interferon injections recently, and there were no other medication changes.

Examination

She was afebrile. Her cranial nerve exam revealed a relative afferent pupillary defect in the right eye, as well as optic nerve pallor without obvious swelling of the optic nerve head. Her motor strength testing was normal, but her tone was more spastic in the legs compared to the previous examination. Her vibration sensation was decreased from previous testing. Her gait was unsteady and mildly spastic but she did not require a walking aid. However, she was unable to complete the tandem gait due to imbalance. Her reflexes were 3^+ throughout, with down-going toes bilaterally.

Investigations

The patient's complete blood count and urinalysis were normal. A brain MRI with and without gadolinium showed a new enhancing lesion in the left periventricular white matter when compared to the previous scan (Figure 5.2).

Outcome

There is clear evidence of ongoing disease activity despite reported adherence to therapy. She was negative for the presence of John Cunningham virus (JCV) antibodies and elected to transition to natalizumab, on which she has done well. She has remained negative on repeat JCV antibody testing, and her brain MRIs have remained stable.

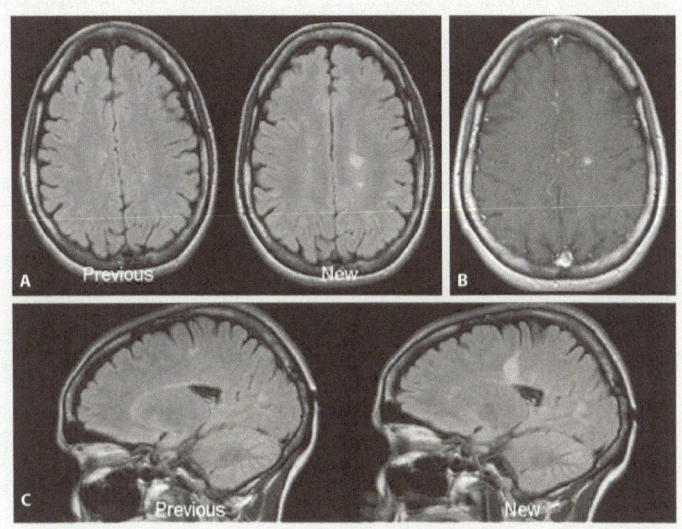

Figure 5.2 Brain MRI with and without gadolinium in a patient with established multiple sclerosis. (**A**) Previous and new axial FLAIR sequences of an MRI brain demonstrating a large new lesion in the left hemisphere. (**B**) T1 MRI with gadolinium demonstrating the same lesion with active enhancement. (**C**) Previous and new sagittal FLAIR MRI demonstrating a large new periventricular lesion.

Discussion

The initial challenge for those on established MS treatments with new symptoms is to determine whether the presentation represents a true treatment failure. With the advent of new disease-modifying therapies (DMTs) in recent years, concepts of breakthrough disease and treatment failure have begun to be re-evaluated. Whereas neurologists were previously willing to accept some degree of ongoing disease activity without switching DMTs, the current goal of treatment is increasingly 'no evidence of disease activity' (NEDA) [1]. From a clinical standpoint, this can most commonly be interpreted as an absence of new clinical relapses or new lesions on MRI, but may also be broadened to include disease progression, neuropsychological outcomes, fatigue, and even quality of life measures [2].

Previously, many neurologists were willing to accept some degree of ongoing clinical or radiologic disease activity despite treatment, though there were no clear or widely accepted guidelines and the threshold for switching treatments varied among clinicians. This was at least partly due to the small number of DMTs available, several of which were quite similar with regard to mechanism of action. While the individual clinician's threshold still varies, and there is still a lack of clearly defined treatment algorithms, many physicians now routinely accept less disease activity due to the larger variety of available therapies.

This is a distinct paradigm shift from the era when some degree of breakthrough disease was acceptable due to the limited number of 'partially effective' therapies and, therefore, was not necessarily considered a treatment failure. While an absence of disease activity may be a difficult therapeutic goal, the trend signals a willingness of physicians to escalate to more aggressive therapies earlier in the course of the disease with the goal of halting any further disease activity and preventing additional disability accumulation [1].

Evaluating breakthrough disease

In the evaluation of new neurologic symptoms, patients are frequently assessed for disorders that may result in the emergence of previously experienced symptoms, sometimes referred to as pseudo-relapses or pseudo-exacerbations. Fatigue, metabolic dysfunction, or mild infection, such as an upper respiratory or urinary tract infection, are a frequent source of such presentations. Evaluation of new symptoms is variable and may be as simple as a thorough history, or it may necessitate additional imaging and serologic workup.

Magnetic resonance imaging

MRI is often employed in the evaluation of new relapsing MS symptoms. MRI techniques have advanced dramatically over the last few decades with improvements in scan acquisition techniques, better tissue contrast and spatial resolution, and new analysis methods [3]. Several MRI metrics are proving to be meaningful surrogate outcome measures in therapeutic drug trials and may provide insights into risk of disability progression in relapsing MS independent of clinical relapses [4]. Furthermore, new lesions early in the treatment course may predict later treatment nonresponse [5] and either new T2 lesions or gadolinium-enhancing T1 lesions during the first year of treatment have been shown to correlate with future disability progression [6–8]. Thus, disease activity as seen on MRI in a patient on immunomodulatory therapy represents a measure of treatment response. Though MRI changes should be viewed in the appropriate clinical context, new T2 or gadolinium-enhancing lesions may warrant initiating a discussion regarding treatment optimization, and in some cases may trigger a treatment change even in the absence of a new overt clinical relapse.

Uhthoff's phenomenon

Many people with MS and other neurological demyelinating disorders experience a worsening of neurologic symptoms associated with overheating. Originally described in 1890, Wilhelm Uhthoff observed a worsening of vision with exercise in patients with optic neuritis [9]. While he associated the phenomenon primarily with exercise, it was later concluded that the etiology was heat. Worsening of a variety of symptoms can be seen with increased body temperature associated with hot weather, exercise, fever, hot tubs, and saunas.

Symptoms related to Uhthoff's phenomenon can initially be difficult to differentiate from true relapses but is essential in order to determine an appropriate intervention. However, a thorough history can usually be enough to recognize the difference. Symptoms related to Uhthoff's phenomenon are typically recurrent, which are stereotyped, short in duration, and reversible, often resolving in minutes to hours by simply resting or removing the inciting insult [10]. The fundamental underlying feature is elevated core body temperature [11]. Through normalization of body temperature, symptoms typically resolve completely [9].

Where available, aquatic therapy can be used to help heat-sensitive individuals to exercise in an appropriate environment. Cooling vests can also allow patients who would otherwise be restricted to air-conditioned environments to partake in outdoor activities.

Adherence

In this patient, where there is clear evidence of ongoing disease activity with new symptoms and new MRI lesions, additional consideration should be given to adherence to current therapy. Even the best medications are unlikely to be effective if not administered appropriately. Any underlying cause of decreased adherence should be determined, as it will likely impact the choice of second-line treatment. For example, if someone is not taking interferon due to fear of needles, it is unlikely that more frequent interferon or glatiramer acetate injections will fare any better.

There are a variety of reasons for medication nonadherence. A common cause is a perceived lack of efficacy [12]. Many patients perceive that treatment is ineffective when their current symptoms do not resolve. Pseudorelapses can also contribute to this perception. Since the currently available therapies are not cures and are only intended to prevent additional disease activity, it is important to set reasonable expectations when discussing treatment options.

All medications have adverse effects. While some adverse effects can simply be an annoyance, others, such as cardiac effects or progressive multifocal leukoencephalopathy, can actually be life threatening. Either way, they can all affect quality of life and are a major reason for nonadherence. With the injectable therapies, injection site reactions and needle fatigue can also contribute [13].

In some cases, treatments may be a 'victim of their own success.' In patients who feel well when on treatment or who go several years without evidence of relapses, there may a perception that they no longer need treatment [14]. This can be especially problematic in individuals who had few overt symptoms to begin with. Conversely, perceived benefits of treatment can also actually improve adherence [15].

Cost, lack of insurance or ability to meet insurance deductibles or copays can also affect the ability to continue, or in some cases even start, medications. Many of the pharmaceutical companies that manufacture MS therapies have financial assistance programs to mitigate this problem, but it continues to be an obstacle for some patients in certain countries.

Strategies to improve patient adherence include setting realistic expectations, addressing adverse events, dealing with injection anxiety where applicable, and developing a successful provider–patient relationship [16].

Switching therapies

There may be several reasons to consider a change in therapy. Commonly, these include inability to tolerate the initial medication, detection of antibodies (either neutralizing or JCV antibodies), and unacceptable treatment response [17]. Both clinical relapses and MRI features are commonly used to establish treatment response, but a decision to switch therapies should be placed in the clinical context. It is a relatively easy decision to transition to another treatment in those with highly active disease, but in patients with a single relapse or a single MRI lesion after several years of stability, a change in therapy may not have any long-term benefit [18]. Once a decision to change therapy has been made, there are no established or widely accepted treatment algorithms when choosing a second-line DMT. It is often a highly individual choice, requiring input from both the physician and the patient, with significant time spent educating the patient about their treatment options. Efficacy, adverse effects, route of administration, long-term risks, and risk aversion all need to be considered. Often the right medication is the one the patient will take consistently.

Clinical pearls

- In the event of new clinical symptoms in established multiple sclerosis, it is highly important to distinguish between 'true' relapse and pseudo-relapse, as seen with Uhthoff's phenomenon.
- As with many disorders, medication adherence is a major consideration in those with ongoing disease activity. A thorough assessment of adherence and strategies to encourage adherence should be employed whenever necessary.
- There are many factors to consider when switching therapies. Both physician and patient play a role. Education regarding efficacy, adverse effects, and long-term management goals can promote adherence and set reasonable expectations.

References

1   Rotstein DL, Healy BC, Malik MT, Chitnis T, Weiner HL. Evaluation of no evidence of disease activity in a 7-year longitudinal multiple sclerosis cohort. *JAMA Neurol*. 2015;72:152-158.

2   Stangel M, Penner IK, Kieseier BC. Defining the new end point for multiple sclerosis treatment. *JAMA Neurol*. 2014;71:1056-1057.

3   Barkhof F, Simon JH, Fazekas F, et al. MRI monitoring of immunomodulation in relapse-onset multiple sclerosis trials. *Nat Rev Neurol*. 2012;8:13-21.

4   Sormani MP, Li DK, Bruzzi P, et al. Combined MRI lesions and relapses as a surrogate for disability in multiple sclerosis. *Neurology*. 2011;77:1684-1690.

5   Kinkel RP, Simon JH, O'Connor P, Hyde R, Pace A. Early MRI activity predicts treatment nonresponse with intramuscular interferon beta-1a in clinically isolated syndrome. *Mult Scler Relat Disord*. 2014;3:712-719.

6   Prosperini L, Gallo V, Petsas N, Borriello G, Pozzilli C. One-year MRI scan predicts clinical response to interferon beta in multiple sclerosis. *Eur J Neurol*. 2009;16:1202-1209.

7   Rio J, Comabella M, Montalban X. Predicting responders to therapies for multiple sclerosis. *Nat Rev Neurol*. 2009;5:553-560.

8   Rudick RA, Lee JC, Simon J, Ransohoff RM, Fisher E. Defining interferon beta response status in multiple sclerosis patients. *Ann Neurol*. 2004;56:548-555.

9   Uhthoff W. Untersuchungen uber die bei der multiplen Herdsklerose vorkommenden Augenstorungen. *Arch Psychiatr Nervenkr*. 1890;21:303-420. German.

10   Frohman TC, Davis SL, Beh S, Greenberg BM, Remington G, Frohman EM. Uhthoff's phenomena in MS--clinical features and pathophysiology. *Nat Rev Neurol*. 2013;9:535-540.

11   Fromont A, Benatru I, Gignoux L, Couvreur G, Confavreux C, Moreau T. [Long-lasting and isolated Uhthoff's phenomenon after effort preceding multiple sclerosis]. *Rev Neurol (Paris)*. 2010;166:61-65. French.

12   Rio J, Porcel J, Tellez N, et al. Factors related with treatment adherence to interferon beta and glatiramer acetate therapy in multiple sclerosis. *Mult Scler*. 2005;11:306-309.

13   Clerico M, Barbero P, Contessa G, Ferrero C, Durelli L. Adherence to interferon-beta treatment and results of therapy switching. *J Neurol Sci*. 2007;259:104-108.

14   Cohen B. Adherence to disease-modifying therapy for multiple sclerosis. *Int J MS Care*. 2006;(suppl):32-37.

15   Turner AP, Kivlahan DR, Sloan AP, Haselkorn JK. Predicting ongoing adherence to disease modifying therapies in multiple sclerosis: utility of the health beliefs model. *Mult Scler*. 2007;13:1146-1152.

16   Costello K, Kennedy P, Scanzillo J. Recognizing nonadherence in patients with multiple sclerosis and maintaining treatment adherence in the long term. *Medscape J Med*. 2008;10:225.

17   Coyle PK. Switching therapies in multiple sclerosis. *CNS Drugs*. 2013;27:239-247.

18   Healy BC, Glanz BI, Stankiewicz J, Buckle G, Weiner H, Chitnis T. A method for evaluating treatment switching criteria in multiple sclerosis. *Mult Scler*. 2010;16:1483-1489.

Progressive multifocal leukoencephalopathy

Chris Eckstein

History

While out-of-town visiting family, a 54-year-old female previously diagnosed with relapsing-remitting multiple sclerosis (RRMS) presented to
the clinic as a new patient to be evaluated for a recent exacerbation,
manifesting with abrupt onset of constant, mild vertigo, and increasingly frequent falls, with progressive deterioration over the last 6 weeks.
She also had some mild nausea, but denied any emesis or weight loss.
There were no cognitive, personality, or behavioral changes reported.

The patient was originally diagnosed with RRMS 8 years prior to
this presentation, following an acute episode of paraparesis with an
incomplete recovery. She was initially treated with glatiramer acetate
daily for 2 years following the diagnosis, but after an additional exacerbation consisting of worsening paraparesis and incontinence with a
new spinal cord lesion, she was transitioned to natalizumab, on which
she has remained over the last 6 years with no additional exacerbations
or new lesions. She did not know if her John Cunningham virus (JCV)
status had been checked in the last year.

Examination

The patient was afebrile and in no acute distress. Her cognition, attention,
and memory appeared normal, although she had a mild scanning quality
to her speech. Her vision and pupils were normal, but she had marked

© Springer International Publishing Switzerland 2017   43
P.S. Giacomini (ed.), *Case Studies in Multiple Sclerosis*,
DOI 10.1007/978-3-319-31190-6_6

bilateral horizontal end-gaze nystagmus on lateral gaze to either side. She was mildly weak in the legs, but reported this was unchanged from her previous visits. She was also weak in her right arm, with 4/5 strength in the biceps, triceps, wrist extensors, and grip, which she had not previously noticed. There was mild spasticity in her legs. She had moderate ataxia with finger-nose testing on the right and with casual gait. She was not able to tandem, toe, or heel walk. Her reflexes were 3[+] throughout, with down-going toes bilaterally.

Investigations

Routine blood work including complete blood count, metabolic profile, liver function, and urinalysis were normal. Her JCV antibody status was unknown at the time of the visit. An MRI was performed and revealed an irregular hyperintensity in the right pons without active gadolinium enhancement (Figure 6.1). Lumbar puncture demonstrated a mildly elevated cerebrospinal fluid (CSF) white blood cell count and protein, with a positive JCV polymerase chain reaction (PCR) result.

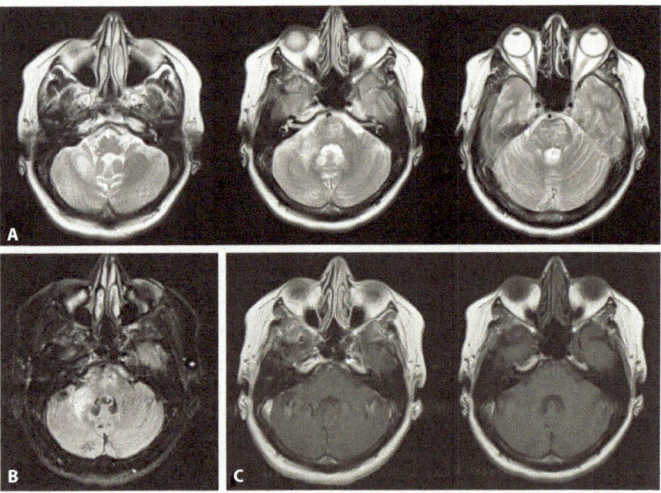

Figure 6.1 (A) T2, (B) FLAIR, and (C) T1 with gadolinium sequences of an MRI brain demonstrating a nonenhancing right pontine lesion later determined to be progressive multifocal leukoencephalopathy.

Outcome

The patient's symptoms had been ongoing for 6 weeks and she was found to have a brainstem lesion with imaging features of progressive multifocal leukoencephalopathy (PML). Due to the high suspicion for the infection, she was admitted and underwent a lumbar puncture with CSF sent for JCV PCR analysis. The JCV PCR test was ultimately positive, confirming a diagnosis of PML. Plasmapheresis was started immediately to accelerate clearance of the natalizumab and she remained stable for several weeks. However, she eventually began to deteriorate and was given pulse steroids for suspected immune reconstitution inflammatory syndrome (IRIS), as repeat imaging revealed expansion of the brainstem lesion (Figure 6.2). Despite all clinical efforts, she died approximately 6 weeks after the PML diagnosis had been confirmed.

Discussion

This case demonstrates some common clinical challenges. First, there is the familiar clinical scenario of a new patient with a prolonged disease

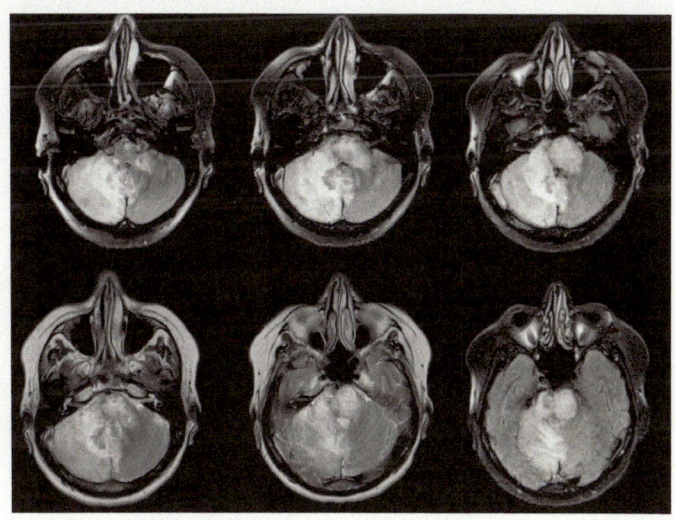

Figure 6.2 T2 sequence of a follow-up MRI brain demonstrating extension of the previously identified right pontine lesion.

and treatment history, for which medical records and documentation is not available at the time of presentation. Without previous imaging for comparison, assessing for the presence of new lesions can be challenging unless there is evidence of gadolinium enhancement. Even then, it is difficult to be certain about an underlying diagnosis in some cases. In this case, records were obtained from her primary neurologist but they did not include her JCV antibody status.

It is significant that the patient's JCV antibody status was not known at the time of the visit. While alternative etiologies should be considered in any person with MS experiencing new symptoms, an additional concern in this case is the presence of a relapse after several years of disease stability while on natalizumab therapy. Given that early detection and diagnosis of PML may lead to improved outcomes [1], a high level of suspicion for JCV infection should be maintained in any case of natalizumab exposure with new neurologic symptoms. While MRI may provide a great deal of insight to an underlying infection [2], lumbar puncture with PCR testing for the presence of JCV DNA is necessary for definitive diagnosis, though there are cases of PML in which the initial JCV PCR was negative due to a low number of viral copies [3]. Thus, a negative JCV PCR should not override a high clinical suspicion of PML in the appropriate clinical context. The presence of JCV activity in the CSF in this patient indicates active infection, which is consistent with a diagnosis of PML, a known complication of natalizumab therapy.

Natalizumab

Natalizumab is a recombinant, humanized monoclonal antibody given as a monthly intravenous infusion for the treatment of RRMS. It targets the α_4 subunit of $\alpha_4\beta_1$ and $\alpha_4\beta_7$ integrins and, as a result, interferes with leukocyte migration across the blood–brain barrier by hindering the interaction between very late antigen (VLA)-4 and vascular endothelial adhesion molecule (VCAM)-1 [4].

Two Phase III clinical trials have shown natalizumab to be a highly effective therapy for RRMS, demonstrated by a variety of clinical endpoints [5,6]. However, there were two cases of PML associated with its use in clinical trials, prompting its withdrawal from the market. It was eventually reintroduced for MS treatment, but a detailed risk–benefit assessment is necessary prior to starting individual treatment. Since its reintroduction, there have been numerous additional cases of PML, which has prompted studies in to risk stratification.

Progressive multifocal leukoencephalopathy

PML, an opportunistic demyelinating encephalopathy due to reactivation of the JCV, was originally identified in patients with severe immunosuppression and is now a well-recognized risk of natalizumab therapy. It is also increasingly being recognized as a potential complication of other immunomodulatory therapies used for MS and has been reported in patients taking fingolimod and dimethyl fumarate, though the significance of the association is still under investigation. The virus itself is common and found in a majority of the population, but only becomes active in those with decreased immune defenses. Additional risk factors for reactivation include prior use of immunosuppression and prolonged duration of natalizumab use [7].

Unfortunately, symptoms of active infection can vary widely, frequently mimicking typical MS exacerbations, though it is usually thought to progress more slowly than classic MS relapses. Common presentations of PML include problems with coordination, cognitive deficits, paresis, and speech disturbance [8].

Aside from the JCV DNA PCR analysis, additional diagnostic clues can be identified on a brain MRI. It can sometimes be difficult to distinguish from MS lesions, especially in those with a high T2 lesion burden, but PML is most evident as a subcortical hyperintense region on T2 and FLAIR imaging. These can sometimes be subtle, with a corresponding hypointense lesion on T1 sequences. Gadolinium enhancement is uncommon [2,9].

Once the diagnosis is established (or highly suspected), treatment options are unfortunately limited. As there are no effective antivirals currently available for PML, the most effective course of treatment involves reversing the immune-compromised state. In the case of natalizumab, the initial step is typically plasmapheresis to accelerate clearance of the monoclonal antibody [10]. However, this may result in a subsequent influx of inflammatory cells into the central nervous system, resulting in IRIS, which then may result in additional complications, disability, or death [11]. While there is currently no widely agreed upon therapeutic approach to PML-related IRIS, multiple centers are actively investigating potential treatment strategies [12].

Natalizumab-associated PML has a mortality rate of approximately 20%, with survivors often left with some degree of neurologic impairment. Additional indicators of poor prognosis include delayed time to diagnosis, high JCV DNA load in the CSF, MS disease duration, gadolinium enhancement on MRI, and a history of previous immunosuppression [13].

Clinical pearls

- Due to the risk of PML, health care providers should have a low threshold for assessing for active PML infection in breakthrough disease in those on, or who have recently discontinued, natalizumab, including evaluation with MRI and lumbar puncture.
- In those treated with natalizumab, as well as other medications with increased PML risk, close monitoring of JCV antibody status should be maintained.
- Patients with negative JCV antibody testing should be retested periodically while on treatment. Many centers are now testing every 6 months due to the risk of negative-to-positive conversion. Additionally, some centers are performing surveillance MRIs more frequently than the typical yearly MRI, though there are no standard guidelines for its use at this point.
- A negative JCV DNA PCR should not negate a high clinical suspicion for PML. Due to the inability of some assays to detect below certain viral loads, negative testing is possible despite active infection. As such, it may be appropriate to initiate plasmapheresis in the setting of a negative PCR.

References

1 Cordioli C, De Rossi N, Rasia S, Lodoli G, Capra R. Early detection and favourable outcome of natalizumab-related progressive multifocal leukoencephalopathy (PML) in two multiple sclerosis patients. *Neurol Sci*. 2015;36:489-491.

2 Wattjes MP, Barkhof F. Diagnosis of natalizumab-associated progressive multifocal leukoencephalopathy using MRI. *Curr Opin Neurol*. 2014;27:260-270.

3 Babi M-A, Pendlebury W, Braff S, Waheed W. JC Virus PCR detection Is not infallible: a fulminant case of progressive multifocal leukoencephalopathy with false-negative cerebrospinal fluid studies despite progressive clinical course and radiological findings. *Case Rep Neurol Med*. 2015;2015:4.

4 Rudick RA, Sandrock A. Natalizumab: alpha 4-integrin antagonist selective adhesion molecule inhibitors for MS. *Expert Rev Neurother*. 2004;4:571-580.

5 Polman CH, O'Connor PW, Havrdova E, Hutchinson M, Kappos L, Miller DH, et al. A randomized, placebo-controlled trial of natalizumab for relapsing multiple sclerosis. *N Engl J Med*. 2006;354:899-910.

6 Rudick RA, Stuart WH, Calabresi PA, et al. Natalizumab plus interferon beta-1a for relapsing multiple sclerosis. *N Engl J Med*. 2006;354:911-923.

7 Bloomgren G, Richman S, Hotermans C, et al. Risk of natalizumab-associated progressive multifocal leukoencephalopathy. *N Engl J Med*. 2012;366:1870-1880.

8 Engsig FN, Hansen A-BE, Omland LH, et al. Incidence, clinical presentation, and outcome of progressive multifocal leukoencephalopathy in HIV-infected patients during the highly active antiretroviral therapy era: a nationwide cohort study. *J Infect Dis*. 2009;199:77-83.

9 Sahraian MA, Radue EW, Eshaghi A, Besliu S, Minagar A. Progressive multifocal leukoencephalopathy: a review of the neuroimaging features and differential diagnosis. *Eur J Neurol*. 2012;19:1060-1069.

10 Khatri BO, Man S, Giovannoni G, et al. Effect of plasma exchange in accelerating natalizumab clearance and restoring leukocyte function. *Neurology*. 2009;72:402-409.

11 Rushing EJ, Liappis A, Smirniotopoulos JD, et al. Immune reconstitution inflammatory syndrome of the brain: case illustrations of a challenging entity. *J Neuropathol Exp Neurol*. 2008;67:819-827.

12 Giacomini PS, Rosenberg A, Metz I, Araujo D, Arbour N, Bar-Or A; MIMSTAPI group. Maraviroc and JCvirus-associated immune reconstitution inflammatory syndrome. *N Engl J Med*. 2014; 370:486-488.

13 Clifford DB, De Luca A, Simpson DM, Arendt G, Giovannoni G, Nath A. Natalizumab-associated progressive multifocal leukoencephalopathy in patients with multiple sclerosis: lessons from 28 cases. *Lancet Neurol*. 2010;9:438-446.

Induction therapy

Chris Eckstein

History

A 42-year-old male with a 15-month history of relapsing-remitting multiple sclerosis (RRMS) diagnosed after an episode of optic neuritis presented to the emergency department due to new acute onset of right hemiparesis and paresthesias starting a few hours prior to presentation. After his initial optic neuritis he was found to have multiple lesions consistent with demyelination without enhancement on his MRI of the brain, as well as oligoclonal bands in his cerebrospinal fluid (CSF). He received intravenous (IV) methylprednisolone, with incomplete recovery of his vision. He was started on maintenance injectable therapy.

His disease course has been complicated by multiple exacerbations. Over the last few months, he experienced separate episodes of new gait impairment, bilateral leg weakness and sensory loss, bladder incontinence, and sexual dysfunction. Residual symptoms have persisted after each exacerbation and he now requires a cane while walking. After his first relapse on treatment, his primary neurologist transitioned him to natalizumab. He has recently completed his ninth infusion and had at least two relapses while on treatment, without missing any infusions.

His current symptoms began a few hours prior to his presentation to the emergency department and are progressing. He is concerned that he needs to be switched to another therapy due to his frequent relapses.

© Springer International Publishing Switzerland 2017
P.S. Giacomini (ed.), *Case Studies in Multiple Sclerosis*,
DOI 10.1007/978-3-319-31190-6_7

Examination

He was afebrile and in no acute distress. His speech had a mild scanning quality and he had occasional word-finding difficulty. There was red color desaturation and a relative afferent pupillary defect in the left eye. His strength testing showed power 5/5 in the left arm, 4/5 throughout the left leg, 3/5 in the right triceps, wrist extensors, and hip flexor, and 2/5 with right ankle dorsiflexion. He had spasticity in both legs and his right arm. There was reduced vibration and pinprick distally, with a sensory level at approximately C6. His reflexes were brisk throughout with clonus in both ankles. Toes were upgoing bilaterally.

Investigations

Due to the exam findings, he was admitted for additional evaluation. His complete blood count (CBC), metabolic profile, urinalysis, and vitamin B_{12} levels were normal. His aquaporin-4 antibody and John Cunningham virus (JCV) antibody status were previously negative. He underwent a brain and spine MRI with and without gadolinium that showed multiple demyelinating lesions throughout the brain and spinal cord. There was a new enhancing juxtacortical lesion in the left hemisphere (Figure 7.1).

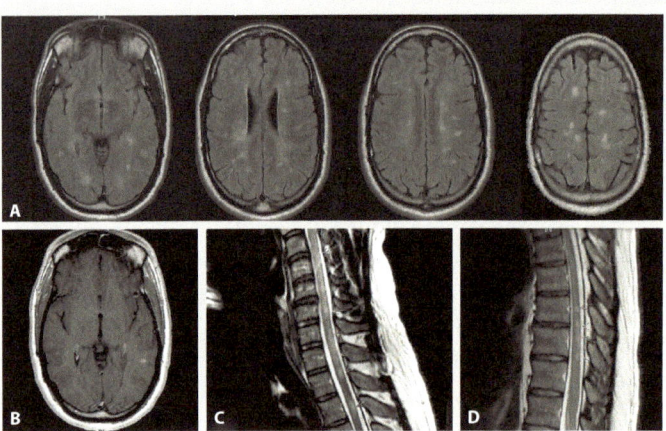

Figure 7.1 The patient's admission MRI showing numerous (A) FLAIR lesions; (B) a new small left enhancing lesion; (C) multiple cervical and (D) lower thoracic spine T2 lesions.

Outcome

This patient tested negative for natalizumab neutralizing antibodies (NAbs). However, this presentation was the third relapse while on natalizumab and he clearly had numerous lesions with a new enhancing lesion on MRI. He received IV methylprednisolone for the new hemiparesis with significant improvement. He then underwent pre-testing for alemtuzumab and eventually transitioned from natalizumab to alemtuzumab. He received an initial alemtuzumab cycle 2 months after his final natalizumab infusion and is, thus far, stable.

Discussion

Patients with multiple exacerbations or new lesions within a short time frame often present a challenge to the clinician. As many of the traditional first-line therapies have significant lag in therapeutic benefit after initiation, choosing an initial therapy can potentially have a marked effect on disability accumulation. Early intervention with disease-modifying agents is thought to delay disability in patients with MS and clinically isolated syndrome [1,2]. Though it is currently not possible to match patients to their optimal treatment, by identifying those with evidence of highly active MS, healthcare providers may be able to employ a more aggressive treatment approach and possibly impact patient outcomes with regards to disability and quality of life.

Highly active multiple sclerosis

Although some degree of disability accumulation can be expected in almost all patients with MS, the rate of disability accumulation is highly variable [3]. However, there appears to be a subset of patients in which the disease progresses at an accelerated rate. Though used inconsistently, the term 'malignant MS' has traditionally been used to refer to a disease course in which patients accumulate disability rapidly. Specifically, they require the use of an assistive device for ambulation (Expanded Disability Status Scale [EDSS] 6.0 or greater) within 5 years of disease onset [4]. Additional definitions have been proposed, including EDSS of 6.0 or greater before the age of 40 and transition to secondary progressive MS (SPMS) within 3 years of relapsing disease onset [5].

Clinical features suggestive of malignant MS include male gender, older age of onset, and presence of a smoking history. Motor symptoms as the initial clinical presentation also suggest more active disease [5,6]. Although there are few studies directly addressing MRI in malignant MS, some MRI findings can suggest more aggressive disease or poor treatment response. For instance, several studies have shown that the development of new T2 lesions or gadolinium-enhancing T1 lesions during the first year of treatment correlate with disability progression [7,8]. Additionally, a higher number of baseline spinal cord lesions on MRI predicts a worse clinical outcome and a higher number of subsequent relapses [9].

Escalation and induction therapy in multiple sclerosis

One of the primary goals in MS treatment is prevention of irreversible neurologic disability. When considering a treatment approach for individual patients with MS, one of the early decisions is whether to use escalation therapy or induction therapy [10].

The most common therapeutic strategy in MS, escalation therapy, typically involves starting with safer medications and escalating to more aggressive and/or riskier agents only when there is evidence that the first-line agents are not controlling disease activity. This strategy necessitates predefined criteria at which a treatment escalation will occur. Additionally, a change to second- or third-line therapy should not be delayed, as irreversible or severe disability may occur [11]. To ensure timely escalation, a standardized approach to the patient evaluation is required to detect treatment failure promptly. Any time that a change in treatment is made, a new baseline should be established, both through exam and MRI. The goal of escalation is to progress through levels of treatment until disease control is achieved [12].

Numerous escalation treatment algorithms have been proposed. However, as additional agents are developed, it is more difficult to reach a consensus. The evidence also becomes more sparse further up the escalation hierarchy because it is difficult to perform large trials on every possible transition or drug combination [12].

Alternatively, induction therapy may be a more appropriate option for some patients, notably those with very active or aggressive disease.

The idea is to 'reset' the immune system. Typical induction strategies involve the minimum effective exposure to intensive immunosuppression to impart disease control, followed by long-term maintenance therapy with a safer or better tolerated agent [11]. This is a common approach in other autoimmune diseases and malignancies.

The most studied induction agent in MS is mitoxantrone, a synthetic anthracenedione derivative with potent immunomodulatory effects currently Food and Drug Administration (FDA)-approved for use in RRMS and SPMS [13]. It is effective in reducing relapses and slowing progression but, due to potential cardiotoxicity and leukemia risk, is limited to a total cumulative dose of $140\,mg/m^2$ [14–16]. Because it was the only available potent immunosuppressant approved for use in MS for several years, mitoxantrone has been evaluated to a greater extent than newer agents. It has been studied as an induction agent with follow-up maintenance therapies consisting of either interferon-beta or glatiramer acetate. In both trials, the induction groups had lower relapse rates and fewer gadolinium-enhancing lesions on MRI than those who were started directly on maintenance therapy without previous induction [17,18].

A newer induction therapy for MS that deserves consideration is alemtuzumab, a humanized monoclonal antibody targeting CD52, a cell-surface marker found on a variety of immune cells [19,20]. It results in rapid, long-lasting depletion of circulating B and T lymphocytes, followed by a slow repopulation from unaffected hematopoietic precursor cells [21,22]. It has demonstrated a significant relapse reduction compared to interferon beta-1a [23,24]. Due to this prolonged repopulation and efficacy, alemtuzumab could be an ideal induction agent. However, it has yet to be studied with a maintenance drug, so there are several unknowns that need to be investigated with this approach. In fact, due to some of its potential risks, such as secondary autoimmunity with thyroid disease, immune thrombocytopenic purpura, and glomerular basement membrane disease, it is still unclear when to readminister alemtuzumab after the initial two annual cycles [25].

Both escalation and induction strategies can be appropriate in the treatment of RRMS and the choice primarily depends on the early course of the disease. Currently, escalation therapy is the predominant treatment approach. However, as newer monoclonal and cytotoxic therapies emerge, the role of induction therapy will likely expand.

Neutralizing antibodies

This patient has experienced several exacerbations while on natalizumab. Although it did not occur in this case, in others experiencing this scenario, NAbs may develop. Natalizumab NAbs can develop early after starting treatment and can be seen transiently in over half of all natalizumab-treated patients after 6 months of treatment [26]. Those with persistently positive NAbs (6%) can have reduced natalizumab concentrations and decreased efficacy. They may also have more frequent hypersensitivity reactions [27]. Due to the transient nature of NAbs, there is insufficient evidence to recommend routine testing in all patients treated with natalizumab.

Clinical pearls

- Clinical features that may correlate with a more aggressive disease course include male gender, older age of onset, history of smoking, and motor symptoms at initial presentation [5,6].
- While escalation therapy may be appropriate for the majority of patients with RRMS, an induction approach may be beneficial in those with aggressive or 'malignant' MS.
- Persistent natalizumab NAbs may result in decreased treatment efficacy and increased adverse events [27].

References

1 Kinkel RP, Kollman C, O'Connor P, et al. IM interferon beta-1a delays definite multiple sclerosis 5 years after a first demyelinating event. *Neurology*. 2006;66:678-684.

2 Kappos L, Freedman MS, Polman CH, et al. Effect of early versus delayed interferon beta-1b treatment on disability after a first clinical event suggestive of multiple sclerosis: a 3-year follow-up analysis of the BENEFIT study. *Lancet*. 2007;370:389-397.

3 Confavreux C, Vukusic S. Natural history of multiple sclerosis: a unifying concept. *Brain*. 2006;129:606-616.

4 DeLuca GC, Ramagopalan SV, Herrera BM, Dyment DA, Lincoln MR, Montpetit A, et al. An extremes of outcome strategy provides evidence that multiple sclerosis severity is determined by alleles at the HLA-DRB1 locus. *Proc Natl Acad Sci U S A*. 2007;104:20896-20901.

5 Menon S, Shirani A, Zhao Y, Oger J, Traboulsee A, Freedman MS, et al. Characterising aggressive multiple sclerosis. *J Neurol Neurosurg Psychiatry*. 2013;84:1192-1198.

6 Gholipour T, Healy B, Baruch NF, Weiner HL, Chitnis T. Demographic and clinical characteristics of malignant multiple sclerosis. *Neurology*. 2011;76:1996-2001.

7 Prosperini L, Gallo V, Petsas N, Borriello G, Pozzilli C. One-year MRI scan predicts clinical response to interferon beta in multiple sclerosis. *Eur J Neurol*. 2009;16:1202-1209.

8 Rio J, Comabella M, Montalban X. Predicting responders to therapies for multiple sclerosis. *Nat Rev Neurol*. 2009;5:553-560.

9 Cordonnier C, de Seze J, et al. Prospective study of patients presenting with acute partial transverse myelopathy. *J Neurol*. 2003;250:1447-1452.

10 Comi G. Induction vs. escalating therapy in multiple sclerosis: practical implications. *Neurol Sci*. 2008;29(suppl 2):S253-S255.

11 Edan G, Le Page E. Induction therapy for patients with multiple sclerosis: why? When? How? *CNS Drugs*. 2013;27:403-409.

12 Rieckmann P. Concepts of induction and escalation therapy in multiple sclerosis. *J Neurol Sci*. 2009;277(suppl 1):S42-S45.

13 Scott LJ, Figgitt DP. Mitoxantrone: a review of its use in multiple sclerosis. *CNS Drugs*. 2004;18:379-396.

14 Edan G, Miller D, Clanet M, et al. Therapeutic effect of mitoxantrone combined with methylprednisolone in multiple sclerosis: a randomised multicentre study of active disease using MRI and clinical criteria. *J Neurol Neurosurg Psychiatry*. 1997;62:112-118.

15 Millefiorini E, Gasperini C, Pozzilli C, et al. Randomized placebo-controlled trial of mitoxantrone in relapsing-remitting multiple sclerosis: 24-month clinical and MRI outcome. *J Neurol*. 1997;244:153-159.

16 Le Page E, Leray E, Edan G, French Mitoxantrone Safety G. Long-term safety profile of mitoxantrone in a French cohort of 802 multiple sclerosis patients: a 5-year prospective study. *Mult Scler*. 2011;17:867-875.

17 Edan G, Comi G, Le Page E, et al. Mitoxantrone prior to interferon beta-1b in aggressive relapsing multiple sclerosis: a 3-year randomised trial. *J Neurol Neurosurg Psychiatry*. 2011;82:1344-1350.

18 Vollmer T, Panitch H, Bar-Or A, et al. Glatiramer acetate after induction therapy with mitoxantrone in relapsing multiple sclerosis. *Mult Scler*. 2008;14:663-670.

19 Xia MQ, Tone M, Packman L, Hale G, Waldmann H. Characterization of the CAMPATH-1 (CDw52) antigen: biochemical analysis and cDNA cloning reveal an unusually small peptide backbone. *Eur J Immunol*. 1991;21:1677-1684.

20 Ginaldi L, De Martinis M, Matutes E, et al. Levels of expression of CD52 in normal and leukemic B and T cells: correlation with in vivo therapeutic responses to Campath-1H. *Leuk Res*. 1998;22:185-191.

21 Hu Y, Turner MJ, Shields J, et al. Investigation of the mechanism of action of alemtuzumab in a human CD52 transgenic mouse model. *Immunology*. 2009;128:260-270.

22 Wiendl H, Kieseier B. Multiple sclerosis: reprogramming the immune repertoire with alemtuzumab in MS. *Nat Rev Neurol*. 2013;9:125-126.

23 Coles AJ, Twyman CL, Arnold DL, et al. Alemtuzumab for patients with relapsing multiple sclerosis after disease-modifying therapy: a randomised controlled phase 3 trial. *Lancet*. 2012;380:1829-1839.

24 Cohen JA, Coles AJ, Arnold DL, et al. Alemtuzumab versus interferon beta 1a as first-line treatment for patients with relapsing-remitting multiple sclerosis: a randomised controlled phase 3 trial. *Lancet*. 2012;380:1819-1828.

25 Coles AJ. Alemtuzumab treatment of multiple sclerosis. *Semin Neurol*. 2013;33:66-73.

26 Vennegoor A, Rispens T, Strijbis EM, et al. Clinical relevance of serum natalizumab concentration and anti-natalizumab antibodies in multiple sclerosis. *Mult Scler*. 2013;19:593-600.

27 Calabresi PA, Giovannoni G, Confavreux C, et al. The incidence and significance of anti-natalizumab antibodies: results from AFFIRM and SENTINEL. *Neurology*. 2007;69:1391-1403.

Primary Progressive
Multiple Sclerosis

Diagnosing primary progressive multiple sclerosis

Scott D. Newsome

History

A 56-year-old man with a history of asthma and anxiety presented for further evaluation of his ongoing neurological decline. He reported being in good neurological health until a few years ago, when he developed left hand clumsiness followed by some difficulty ambulating due to fatigable weakness in his left leg. He noticed that his left leg would become weak while walking long distances but then would improve after resting. These symptoms prompted neurophysiological studies that demonstrated mild bilateral median neuropathies at the wrist, which was thought to be contributing to his hand symptoms. Lower extremity neurophysiological testing did not reveal a polyneuropathy, myopathy, or radiculopathy. He subsequently underwent a lumbar spine MRI for his ambulation difficulties that demonstrated some degenerative disk disease, but no spinal stenosis or nerve root compression.

The patient reported that from the initial onset of his left hand symptoms, he has noticed progressive worsening in not only his dexterity, but also strength on his left side. Over the last few years, he noticed progressive upper left arm and left leg involvement, which has led to an unstable gait at times. His symptoms are much worse towards the end of the day and he gets fatigable weakness quite easily. Over the last several months, he developed a left foot drop and left arm tightness. He had a fall 6 months ago due to tripping over a rug and has had multiple

© Springer International Publishing Switzerland 2017

P.S. Giacomini (ed.), *Case Studies in Multiple Sclerosis*,
DOI 10.1007/978-3-319-31190-6_8

near-falls due to his foot drop. He has not experienced any bladder or bowel issues, bulbar dysfunction, diplopia, or vision loss.

Examination

The patient's general medical exam had no significant findings, except for vasomotor changes in his left hand and foot. His neurologic exam was most notable for nystagmus in left horizontal gaze and reported horizontal diplopia when looking left. There was mild spasticity in the left upper and lower extremities, with left upper extremity weakness (4/5 strength for triceps, biceps, wrist extensors, finger extensors, and hand grip), left lower extremity weakness (4/5 strength in hip flexors and ankle dorsiflexors), and hyperreflexia of the left upper and lower extremities, with an extensor plantar response on left. He also had decreased fine finger movements and foot tapping on the left and his gait evaluation had a left hemiparetic element with mild left circumduction and left hip hiking. There was moderate difficulty with tandem walking, inability to heel-walk on the left, and inability to stand on his left leg independently for 5 seconds.

Investigations

The patient's routine laboratory studies were unremarkable and his erythrocyte sedimentation rate, C-reactive protein, vitamin B_{12}, methylmalonic acid, copper, ceruloplasmin, zinc, angiotensin-converting enzyme, neuromyelitis optica immunoglobulin (NMO-Ig) G, HIV, Lyme antibodies, rapid plasma reagin, human T-lymphotropic virus 1, antinuclear antibody, anti-dsDNA antibody, anti-RNP antibody, anti-Smith antibody, anti-Ro antibody, anti-La antibody, C3 complement, C4 complement, anti-neutrophilic cytoplasmic antibodies, 65 kDa isoform of glutamic acid decarboxylase (antiGAD65) antibody, collapsin-response mediator protein 5 antibody, and antiphospholipid antibodies were all normal or negative. A brain MRI demonstrated a T2 hyperintense right midbrain lesion and a couple of juxtacortical lesions (Figure 8.1). An MRI of the cervical and thoracic spinal cord demonstrated a T2 hyperintense lesion at C1, T1, T7, and T11 (Figure 8.2). None of the lesions enhanced following the administration of gadolinium on T1-weighted sequences.

An MRI of the lumbar spine demonstrated mild degenerative disc disease. Lumbar puncture revealed no white blood cells, normal protein, normal glucose, negative gram stain, negative viral and fungal studies, normal flow cytometry, negative cytopathology, and the presence of intrathecal antibody production (ie, elevated IgG index at 1.2 [within normal range of 0.2–0.8] and positive oligoclonal bands that were restricted to the cerebrospinal fluid [CSF]).

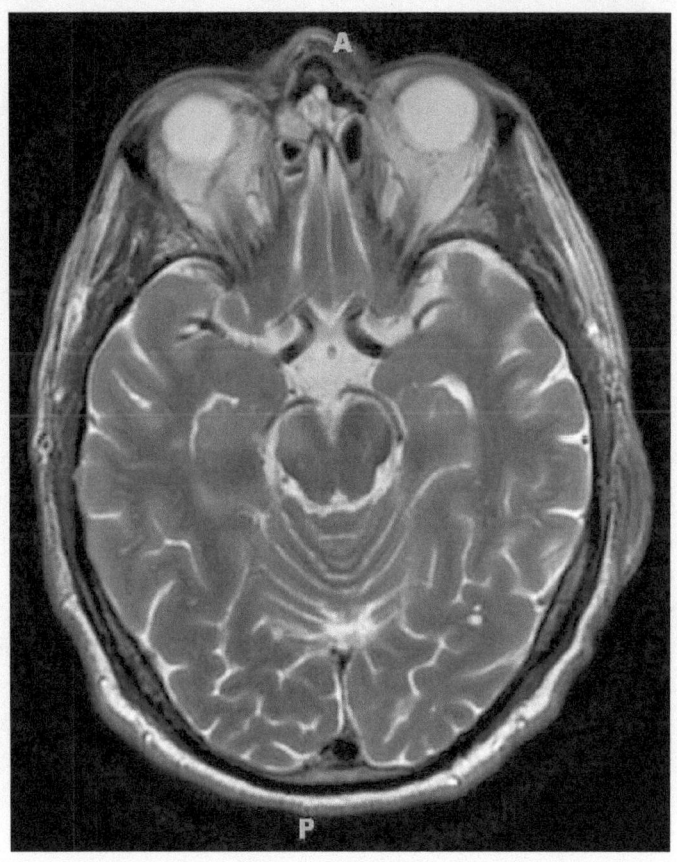

Figure 8.1 Axial T2-weighted sequence of a brain MRI showing a right midbrain lesion.

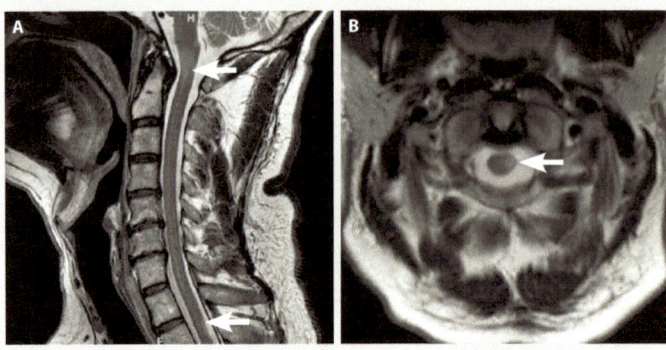

Figure 8.2 MRI of the cervical and thoracic spinal cord. **(A)** Sagittal T2-weighted sequence of a cervical spine MRI showing C1 and T1 lesions. **(B)** Axial T2-weighted sequence of a cervical spine MRI showing a lesion at C1.

Outcome

After reviewing the clinical evolution of slowly progressive neurological deterioration, as well as the patient's imaging, laboratory serologic testing, and CSF results, the patient was diagnosed with primary progressive multiple sclerosis (PPMS).

Discussion

This case illustrates a fairly common presentation of PPMS, which accounts for approximately 10–15% of the MS patient population. PPMS is characterized clinically by progressive worsening of neurological symptoms and function from the onset, without interposed relapses [1]. In fact, this subtype of MS does not have clinical relapses like the relapsing forms of MS. However, patients with PPMS can have amplification or intensification of symptoms throughout the course of a day, as highlighted in the case presented, which can sometimes be mistaken for a relapse. Men are equally as affected with PPMS as women and the typical age at symptom onset is older than 40 years of age. African-Americans appear to have a higher prevalence of PPMS when compared to Caucasians [2,3]. Patients with PPMS have a more rapid accumulation of disability relative to relapsing-remitting MS (RRMS), although being younger and having sensory symptoms at onset appear to be associated with a slower disease progression [4]. Alternatively, motor onset symptoms seem to be associated with a faster disease progression [4].

PPMS classically presents with a progressive myelopathy and gait disorder secondary to leg weakness, spasticity, and impaired coordination. Patients with PPMS typically have fewer gadolinium-enhancing lesions on MRI than relapsing forms of MS and generally greater involvement of the spinal cord than the brain, as illustrated by the case presented. More recent studies have shown that spinal cord atrophy measured at the C2 vertebral level is greater in patients with progressive disease than relapsing disease and that this measure correlates strongly with clinical disability [5]. Gray matter abnormalities have also been identified in PPMS with magnetization transfer ratio imaging, and these changes have been associated with cognitive dysfunction [6]. These findings highlight greater global central nervous system involvement in PPMS.

Histopathological and spinal fluid assessments have consistently demonstrated less overt inflammation in PPMS than other subtypes of MS [7,8]. These findings may suggest that patients with PPMS have less disruption of the blood–brain barrier and more non-inflammatory mechanisms facilitating their disease progression compared to relapsing forms of MS. Moreover, some pathologic studies have suggested that PPMS may represent a primary problem with the oligodendrocyte [7].

The case presented is most consistent with an upper motor neuron syndrome, which in the context of progressive neurological decline without obvious relapses and an MRI demonstrating multifocal white matter lesions, necessitates strong consideration for a PPMS diagnosis. However, there are several conditions that can mimic PPMS that also need to be considered including vitamin B_{12} deficiency, copper deficiency, spinal stenosis, Sjögren's syndrome myelopathy, stiff person syndrome, and primary lateral sclerosis, among others. There is no single diagnostic test for diagnosing PPMS; therefore, diagnostic criteria have been developed that incorporate clinical features supplemented by paraclinical testing.

The revised 2010 McDonald criteria were developed by a panel of MS experts in order to help clinicians determine whether an individual has a specific type of MS or not. The latest criteria requires specific clinical and paraclinical factors to support a diagnosis of PPMS including one year of disease progression, plus two out of three following criteria:

- ≥1 T2 lesions in typical MS regions;
- ≥2 T2 lesions in the spinal cord; or
- intrathecal antibody production (unique CSF oligoclonal bands and/or elevated IgG index) [9].

Ruling out other diseases including those mentioned above is necessary before an official diagnosis of PPMS can be given. As part of excluding other disease processes it is prudent to obtain multiple serological studies as was done in the case presented. It is also extremely important to rule out structural pathology (spinal stenosis) via neuraxial imaging and in some cases hereditary neurodegenerative diseases (hereditary spastic paraparesis) or other rare immune-mediated diseases (stiff person syndrome, CRMP-5 related myelopathy) because these conditions can result in progressive neurological disability.

Despite the recent advances in our understanding of the pathogenesis of MS and the increasing number of available immunomodulating and immunosuppressive therapies to treat MS, there are currently no approved therapies that have proven to impact disability progression in PPMS. However, many clinicians will still recommend starting one of the currently available MS disease-modifying therapies (DMTs) in hopes of decreasing neurological decline in PPMS, especially because there may be a subgroup of patients who respond favorably to these therapies. In a multicenter, randomized, double-blind, placebo controlled study evaluating rituximab (a CD20⁺ B-cell-depleting monoclonal antibody) in patients with PPMS, a subgroup analysis demonstrated that individuals who were <51 years of age and/or who had gadolinium-enhancing lesions on MRI had a significant delay in their confirmed disability progression when compared to placebo [10]. However, the overall study proved to be negative.

A recent clinical trial evaluating ocrelizumab, a related anti-CD20 B-cell-depleting monoclonal antibody, showed that this molecule had a modest effect in slowing progression in PPMS; however, the full results and details from this study have yet to be published. At this juncture, the cornerstone of treatment for PPMS is symptomatic and rehabilitative in nature. Recognition and treatment of ongoing symptoms can greatly improve the quality of life for patients with PPMS. Additionally, lifestyle modifications including exercise in moderation, smoking cessation, and vitamin D supplementation may help impact disease progression.

Clinical pearls

- PPMS accounts for 10–15% of the MS patient population.
- PPMS does not have clinical relapses.
- Men and women are equally affected with PPMS.
- The typical age at symptom onset for PPMS is >40 years of age.
- Older age at symptom onset and motor symptoms present at onset are both associated with a faster disease progression.
- PPMS classically presents with a progressive myelopathy and gait disorder.
- Patients with PPMS have fewer gadolinium-enhancing lesions on MRI than relapsing forms of MS, which supports a greater role of noninflammatory mechanisms for disease progression.
- Patients with PPMS usually have greater spinal cord than brain involvement.
- Revised McDonald criteria for diagnosing PPMS requires at least one year of disease progression plus the following two out of three criteria: ≥1 T2 lesions in typical MS regions; ≥2 T2 lesions in the spinal cord; and/or intrathecal antibody production.
- Currently available DMTs have proven to be ineffective in PPMS which could be the result of a relatively intact blood-brain barrier.
- The cornerstone of treatment for PPMS is symptomatic and rehabilitative in nature, along with lifestyle modifications. These interventions can greatly improve the quality of life for patients with PPMS.

References

1   Lublin F, Reingold SC, Cohen JA, et al. Defining the clinical course of multiple sclerosis: The 2013 revisions. *Neurology* 2014;83;278-286.

2   Koch M, Kingwell E, Rieckmann P, Tremlett H. The natural history of primary progressive multiple sclerosis. *Neurology* 2009;73:1996-2002.

3   Naismith RT, Trinkaus K, Cross AH. Phenotype and prognosis in African-Americans with multiple sclerosis: a retrospective chart review. *Mult Scler.* 2006;12:775-781.

4   Koch MW, Greenfield J, Javizian O, Deighton S, Wall W, Metz LM. The natural history of early versus late disability accumulation in primary progressive MS. *J Neurol Neurosurg Psychiatry.* 2015;86:615-621.

5   Bernitsas E, Bao F, Seraji-Bozorgzad N, et al. Spinal cord atrophy in multiple sclerosis and relationship with disability across clnical phenotypes. *Mult Scler Relat Disord.* 2015;4:47-51.

6   Tur C, Penny S, Khaleeli Z, et al. Grey matter damage and overall cognitive impairment in primary progressive multiple sclerosis. *Mult Scler.* 2011 17:1324-1332.

7   Lucchinetti CF, Brück W, Parisi J, Scheithauer B, Rodriguez M, Lassmann H. Heterogeneity of multiple sclerosis lesions: implications for the pathogenesis of demyelination. *Ann Neurol.* 2000;47:707-717.

8   Iwanowski P, Losy J. Immunological differences between classical phenotypes of multiple sclerosis. *J Neurol Sci.* 2015;349:10-14.

9   Polman CH, Reingold SC, Banwell B, et al. Diagnostic criteria for multiple sclerosis: 2010 revisions to the McDonald criteria. *Ann Neurol.* 2011;69:292-302.

10   Hawker K, O'Connor P, Freedman MS, et al. Rituximab in patients with primary progressive multiple sclerosis: results of a randomized double-blind placebo-controlled multicenter trial. *Ann Neurol.* 2009;66:460-471.

Symptomatic care in primary progressive multiple sclerosis

Scott D. Newsome

History

A 60-year-old woman with a long-standing history of primary progressive multiple sclerosis (PPMS) presented for further evaluation of ongoing lower extremity pain. The patient was diagnosed with PPMS 7 years ago after she presented to a neurologist with progressive gait decline and falls. Her initial work-up revealed findings typical for PPMS, including multifocal demyelinating lesions on MRI (spine more than brain) and an elevated immunoglobulin G (IgG) index within her cerebrospinal fluid. Over the last couple of years, the patient developed an uncomfortable burning sensation in her feet circumferentially. This discomfort is worse at night and does not respond to ibuprofen or acetaminophen. Her foot pain will often prevent her from walking long distances and has become more constant. She no longer attends weekly bingo with her friends and rarely leaves her house in order to limit amplification of her pain.

Examination

The patient's general medical exam had no significant findings. Her straight leg raise test was negative and her foot and ankle range of motion appear normal. Her neurologic exam was most notable for mild spasticity in both lower extremities, bilateral lower extremity weakness (3/5 strength in hip flexors, 4/5 in knee flexors, and 4/5 in ankle dorsiflexors), diffuse hyperreflexia with hyperpredominance of reflexes in

© Springer International Publishing Switzerland 2017   69
P.S. Giacomini (ed.), *Case Studies in Multiple Sclerosis*,
DOI 10.1007/978-3-319-31190-6_9

the lower extremities, extensor plantar responses bilaterally, a T9 sensory level to pinprick and superimposed hyperalgesia to tactile stimuli in both feet circumferentially, and a spastic wide-based gait with bilateral leg circumduction and hip hiking.

Investigations

The patient's routine laboratory studies were unremarkable and basic neuropathy investigations were all normal or negative (complete blood count, vitamin B_{12}, methylmalonic acid, copper, ceruloplasmin, thyroid-stimulating hormone, human immunodeficiency virus, lyme antibodies, rapid plasma reagin, antinuclear antibody, erythrocyte sedimentation rate, C-reactive protein, fasting glucose, glycosylated hemoglobin, serum and urine protein electrophoresis). MRI of the brain, cervical spine, and thoracic spine demonstrated no new or enhancing lesions when compared to images from 3 years earlier. An MRI of the lumbar spine demonstrated mild degenerative disc disease but no spinal stenosis or nerve root compression. Her lower extremity neurophysiological testing did not reveal a large fiber polyneuropathy or radiculopathy. Skin punch biopsy was unremarkable for a small fiber neuropathy.

Outcome

The patient's pain is typical of neuropathic pain that is frequently associated with multiple sclerosis (MS), especially in older patients with progressive forms. As in this case, a thorough assessment and investigation should always be undertaken to exclude rheumatologic and peripheral nerve pathology, as these underlying conditions may require different treatments.

Discussion

This case illustrates a common scenario for individuals with a history of long-standing MS. The demyelination and axonal damage that ensues in MS can occur anywhere in the central nervous system (CNS) and provoke symptoms that vary in severity and duration along with change over time. MS-related symptoms have been associated with a poorer quality of life and have shown to negatively impact patients' autonomy and independence. Moreover, the hidden symptoms, including pain, are among the most disabling and life-altering for individuals with MS [1].

The mean prevalence of pain in MS is greater than 50% and approximately one-third of patients consider pain to be their worst symptom [1–3]. Lower limb pain is seen in 40% of people with MS [4]. There are a number of risk factors associated with pain in MS, including older age, longer disease duration, greater disease severity, progressive forms of MS, and presence of depression [5].

The case presented highlights typical features of neuropathic pain. Neuropathic pain is a primary symptom that occurs in MS as a direct consequence of CNS lesion(s) affecting the somatosensory system. It is thought that ephaptic transmission between denuded axons in the spinal cord and/or the brainstem leads to neuropathic pain [2]. Neuropathic pain can vary in presentation and is often described as burning, tingling, stabbing, shooting, electric shock-like, and/or band-like discomfort. It can be persistent and worse at night, as in the case presented, or intermittent, as seen with trigeminal neuralgia and Lhermitte's sign. Neuropathic pain responds poorly to standard analgesics and often needs a multifaceted approach to help treat it. Unfortunately, neuropathic pain remains underrecognized and, therefore, undertreated [6].

Chronic neuropathic pain is associated with other symptoms including fatigue, insomnia, anxiety, and depression [7]. These various symptoms can worsen or precipitate each other and create a cycle that is difficult to break. As demonstrated in this case, an individual's quality of life can suffer greatly when chronic pain is present as it can limit someone from participating in enjoyable activities and lead to a state of isolation.

Treatment for neuropathic pain requires persistence and often a combination of pharmacological and non-pharmacological interventions. There are several classes of medications that are used to treat neuropathic pain in MS including antidepressants, antiepileptics, antiarrhythmics, topicals, and opioids [3]. Evidence to support their use comes from small clinical trials in MS and trials from other diseases with neuropathic pain. There are a few treatment principles that clinicians can use to help improve MS-related pain medication management:

- start with a low dose and gradually titrate to efficacy;
- if partial pain relief occurs with one drug as monotherapy, a combination of two or more different classes of drugs can often yield better results; and
- in general, when patient is pain-free for 3 months on a treatment regimen, consider a slow taper.

Dysesthetic burning extremity or torso pain is often treated with tricyclic antidepressants (TCAs) such as amitriptyline and nortriptyline. These medications are dosed at night due to their most common side effect of somnolence. In addition, patients may experience a dry mouth, urinary retention, and constipation from their anticholinergic effects. Alternatively, antiepileptic medications can be used. Gabapentin and pregabalin are often used as first-line within this class of medications. Common side effects of these medications include weight gain, dizziness, and somnolence. Carbamazepine is often used when pain is very severe (ie, trigeminal neuralgia) or intractable. This agent is associated with numerous side effects including dizziness, somnolence, hyponatremia, elevated liver enzymes, aplastic anemia, and rash, among others. Serotonin and norepinephrine reuptake inhibitors such as duloxetine and venlafaxine are also used for MS-related neuropathic pain. These medications are often very helpful when there is coexisting depression and/or anxiety. Cannabinoids have been tested for the treatment of pain associated with MS with varying success. Side effects of worsening cognitive dysfunction are the current main limiting factor for using cannabinoid-containing therapies routinely. Opioids are rarely used to treat neuropathic pain because of their nonselective treatment of pain syndromes, along with their high incidence of dependency and undesirable side effects.

Various surgical interventions have been used for medication refractory pain. These interventions are often reserved as a last resort; rhizotomies, neurectomies, myelotomies, and spinal cord stimulator placement.

Several non-pharmacological interventions have been used to treat neuropathic pain including exercise, acupuncture, mindfulness approaches, meditation, and relaxation techniques. These interventions have demonstrated some success in treating MS pain, although further studies are needed to better understand how these treatments alter pain.

The majority of patients with MS will require a multifaceted and multidisciplinary approach to treating their chronic symptoms and disability [8]. Hence, it is important to consider referral to other providers with differing expertise (eg, physical therapy, occupational therapy, pain management) to help optimize a patient's treatment over time.

Clinical pearls

- Pain is considered one of the 'hidden' symptoms of MS and occurs in more than 50% of patients.
- There are a number of risk factors associated with pain in MS including older age, longer disease duration, greater disease severity, progressive forms of MS, and the presence of depression.
- A multifaceted and multidisciplinary approach is needed to treat chronic neuropathic pain in MS.
- There are several classes of medications that can be beneficial in treating neuropathic pain in MS including antidepressants, antiepileptics, antiarrhythmics, and opioids.
- If partial pain relief occurs with one drug as monotherapy, a combination of two or more different classes of drugs can often yield better results.
- Neuropathic pain responds poorly to standard analgesics (ie, ibuprofen, naproxen, and acetaminophen).
- Several non-pharmacological interventions have been used to treat neuropathic pain including exercise, acupuncture, mindfulness approaches, meditation, and relaxation techniques.
- Surgical interventions are reserved for medication refractory pain.
- It is important to involve other providers with differing expertise to help optimize a patient's pain treatment over time.

References

1   Schapiro R. *Managing the Symptoms of Multiple Sclerosis*. 6th edn. New York, New York: Demos Medical Publishing; 2014.

2   Osterberg A, Boivie J, Thuomas KA. Central pain in multiple sclerosis--prevalence and clinical characteristics. *Eur J Pain*. 2005;9:531-542.

3   Solaro C, Uccelli MM. Management of pain in multiple sclerosis: a pharmacological approach. *Nat Rev Neurol*. 2011;7:519-527.

4   Beiske AG, Pedersen ED, Czujko B, Myhr KM. Pain and sensory complaints in multiple sclerosis. *Eur J Neurol*. 2004;11:479-482.

5   O'Connor AB, Schwid SR, Herrmann DN, Markman JD, Dworkin RH. Pain associated with multiple sclerosis: systematic review and proposed classification. *Pain*. 2008;137:96-111.

6   Ehde DM, Osborne TL, Jensen MP. Chronic pain in persons with multiple sclerosis. *Phys Med Rehabil Clin N Am*. 2005;16:503-512.

7   Kalia LV, O'Connor PW. Severity of chronic pain and its relationship to quality of life in multiple sclerosis. *Mult Scler*. 2005;11:322-327.

8   Crayton H, Heyman RA, Rossman HS. A multimodal approach to managing the symptoms of multiple sclerosis. *Neurology*. 2004;63(11 suppl 5):S12-S18.

Secondary Progressive Multiple Sclerosis

Diagnosing secondary progressive multiple sclerosis

Sarah Morrow

History

A 36-year-old woman initially presented to her neurologist for evaluation of diplopia. A subsequent MRI of the brain without gadolinium enhancement revealed evidence of demyelinating lesions in both cerebral hemispheres demonstrating dissemination in space, including two lesions in the brainstem and one in the pons. On further questioning, the patient recalled a transient episode of right arm numbness 8 years earlier that had fully resolved spontaneously after 4 weeks. At the time, the symptoms were mild and not investigated any further. Four months after her neurological assessment, she had an episode consistent with a partial transverse myelitis, specifically bilateral paresthesias that started in her feet and migrated up to the buttock area over a week, and then in to her fingers bilaterally, with positive Lhermitte's sign (electric sensation in back and/or limbs). Her Expanded Disability Severity Scale (EDSS) at this time was 2.5. She was diagnosed with relapsing-remitting multiple sclerosis (RRMS) and started on disease-modifying therapy (DMT).

She remained stable for the next 2 years but then began reporting worsening of her symptoms and increasing fatigue; her EDSS remained stable at 2.5. She did not respond to symptomatic treatment for fatigue. One year later, she had a subacute worsening of gait ataxia.

© Springer International Publishing Switzerland 2017
P.S. Giacomini (ed.), *Case Studies in Multiple Sclerosis*,
DOI 10.1007/978-3-319-31190-6_10

Examination

Upon examination in the clinic, in addition to her previous findings, she now had mild heel-to-shin ataxia, could no longer perform a tandem gait, and her Rhomberg's test (measuring sensory ataxia) was positive. Her EDSS was 3.0. She was treated with high-dose corticosteroids and noted only a partial recovery. Six months later, her EDSS increased to 3.5 with new bilateral temporal pallor, latent left intranuclear ophthalmoplegia, mild spasticity in her legs, and dysmetria in all four limbs without any history or relapses. Neutralizing antibodies to interferon were negative.

One year later, the patient is now 41 years old and her EDSS has increased to 5.5, as she can only walk 100 meters without rest or the use of a cane.

Investigations

An MRI of the brain and cervical spine was performed to investigate her worsening disability and compared to a previous scan done 2 years earlier. The radiologist report stated that there was no significant change in lesion load; however, there was a comment describing diffuse brain atrophy compared to her prior scan.

Outcome

This patient is presenting with neurologic worsening and progression, independent of MS relapses. This evolution is typical of patients transitioning to the secondary progressive phase of MS.

Discussion

Secondary progressive MS (SPMS) is the long-term outcome of all relapsing MS cases and is considered the 'second phase' of the disease. The risk of conversion to SPMS was studied in a population in London, Canada from 1972 to 1984 [1]. This study reported that the risk of conversion to SPMS increased with disease duration, with more than 50% of patients converting after the first decade after MS onset and 90% transitioning to SPMS within 25 years [1]. A more recent cohort study from British Columbia, Canada examined patients with MS from September 1980 to July 2003. By the end of this study, only 35% had converted to SPMS.

Median time to SPMS conversion was 21.4 years (95% confidence interval [CI], 20.6–22.2) at a median age of 53.7 years (95% CI, 53.1–54.3) [2]. This study found that presenting with motor system involvement and male gender were risks for a shorter time/younger age of SPMS onset, while those patients with MS who were younger at disease onset took longer to convert to SPMS, but did so at a younger age [2].

The diagnosis of SPMS is retrospective in nature. Generally, it is made after a history of gradual worsening (progression) in a patient with a history of a relapsing-remitting pattern of disease in the past [3,4]. There may still be minor remissions or plateaus but, overall, the course is that of slow accumulation of disability, generally occurring at a constant rate, independent of the number of relapses and relapse severity. Ongoing relapses may still occur and progression is considered to contribute to an SPMS diagnosis if it is independent of residual disability accumulated from relapses and occurs during the interval between relapses [3,4]. The duration of progression that should be present prior to making an SPMS diagnosis has not been fully defined; however, if the diagnostic criteria for primary progressive MS (PPMS) are extrapolated, duration of progression of clinical disability (separate from that accumulated from relapses) of over 1 year is appropriate [5]. Thus, there is often a transitional phase as the disease evolves from a clinically relapsing pattern of the disease to SPMS and the onset can be subtle. One study found an average delay of 2.9 years between the first clinical assessment suggestive of progressive disease to the final definitive diagnosis of SPMS [6].

There are no known imaging, immunological, or pathological criteria to help determine when a relapsing patient transitions to SPMS. In order to monitor change over time, the EDSS can still be used. In this patient, a change on the EDSS was noted as she progressed over time but it is not always sensitive to change. Other measures have been proposed to help monitor for progression over time, such as the Timed 25-Foot Walk (T25-FW), to predict disability in progressive MS populations [7–9]. Studies have demonstrated that a change of 20% or more on the T25-FW is clinically meaningful [10–12]. Other studies have demonstrated that combining the T25-FW with the Nine-Hole Peg Test (9-HPT) is sensitive to clinically relevant changes [11–13].

Another clinical conundrum is how to manage DMTs in SPMS. The approval of numerous DMTs over the last two decades has dramatically changed the treatment landscape for MS. Currently, there are ten DMTs approved for MS with varying degrees of efficacy for reducing relapse risk and preserving neurological function, but their impact on the progressive phase of the disease has not been conclusively shown. The hallmark of the relapsing stage of MS is acute inflammatory lesions, which can either be clinically silent or associated with overt neurological symptoms (eg, a relapse). Although the mechanism of action between therapies differ, DMTs generally act on reducing new inflammatory lesions and relapses, reducing their frequency and severity. In SPMS, disability is thought to accumulate through different degenerative mechanisms. Whether this neurodegeneration is due to the previous inflammatory stage or begins independently but interacts with the inflammatory response during the relapsing phase remains unclear and controversial [14]. In SPMS, inflammation continues to occur, and is associated with both demyelination and neurodegeneration, but unlike in RRMS, the inflammation is not as strongly related to penetration of the blood–brain barrier [14].

Currently, interferon (IFN) beta-1b is approved for the treatment of SPMS in Europe, based on results of the European Secondary Progressive MS (EU-SPMS) trial [15]. This 36-month study's primary outcome, time to confirmed progression in disability, was significantly better in the IFN beta-1b group when compared to placebo (P=0.0008). However, a follow up North American Secondary Progressive MS (NA-SPMS) trial did not find a significant difference on time to confirmed progression and it is not currently available in North America [16]. Both studies found improvement in clinical relapse rate and MRI outcomes in the treatment group. A reanalysis combining the data from both studies found that the EU-SPMS patients were younger and had MS for a shorter time period prior to inclusion in the study when compared to the NA-SPMS subjects. Further, a higher proportion of patients in the EU-SPMS had relapses and disease activity on the MRI prior to inclusion. This reanalysis suggests IFN beta-1b may be effective in the early 'transitional phase' of SPMS when relapses are still present in the progressive phase [17]. Three smaller studies have also examined the use of IFNs in SPMS: International MS Secondary Progressive Avonex Controlled Trial (IMPACT) with IFN beta-1a (60 mg SC weekly) [18]; Secondary Progressive Efficacy Clinical Trial of Recombinant Interferon beta-1a in MS (SPECTRIMS) with IFN beta-1a (22 μg or 44 μg SC three times weekly) [19]; and the Nordic SPMS Study Group with IFN beta-1a (22 μg SC weekly) [20], all of which were negative.

A Cochrane review included all five of these trials to evaluate the efficacy of IFN beta in SPMS [21]. The authors noted the population was heterogeneous in terms of baseline characteristics, specifically the proportion of patients with superimposed relapses in addition to a progressive course. Overall, the Cochrane review found no decreased risk of progression at 6 months, but did find a significant decrease in the risk of progression sustained at 3 months and risk of developing new relapses. The review concluded that IFN beta does not prevent the development of permanent physical disability in SPMS, but does reduce the risk of relapses and short-term (unsustained) disability [21].

Overall, DMTs are not recommended for use in the treatment of SPMS to slow or halt the accumulation of disability over time. Yet, up to 40% of patients with SPMS continue to have relapses [22]. A recent study demonstrated that most 'post-progression' relapses occurred within 5 years (91.6%) of onset of the progressive phase and that DMT use in the early (transitional) phase of SPMS delayed the time to an EDSS of 6.0 [23]. Thus, it may be reasonable to continue treatment in those early SPMS patients who continue to have superimposed relapses or evidence of ongoing inflammatory activity on MRI.

Mitoxantrone, an antineoplastic medication that suppresses both B- and T-cell proliferation, is approved in Europe and the United States. A 2013 Cochrane review of three trials of mitoxantrone vs. placebo concluded that mitoxantrone is partially efficacious at reducing the risk of progression in all types of MS, including SPMS, over a 2-year period, but did note that the results should be interpreted with caution due to heterogeneity between studies [24]. Also, although no significant adverse events were noted in these trials, longer studies have noted significant cardiac adverse events and risk of leukemia [24].

Clinical pearls

- SPMS is the long-term outcome of all relapsing MS cases and is considered the second phase of the disease.
- The diagnosis of SPMS is retrospective in nature, made after a history of gradual worsening (progression) in a patient with a history of a relapsing remitting pattern of disease.
- There is often a period of transition from a purely relapsing phase of the disease to SPMS.
- There is no clear indication to use currently approved DMTs to slow or halt the slow worsening associated with SPMS. However, relapses still occur in up to 40% of patients with SPMS, especially in the early stages, soon after conversion to SPMS. Thus, treatment with DMTs to prevent ongoing relapse activity in SPMS is a reasonable approach.
- The EDSS is not always sensitive to subtle progression in SPMS. Thus, in addition to the EDSS, another measure should be used to measure progression, such as the T25-FW or the 9-HPT.

References

1   Weinshenker BG, Bass B, Rice GP, et al. The natural history of multiple sclerosis: a geographically based study. I. Clinical course and disability. *Brain*. 1989;112(Pt 1):133-146.
2   Koch M, Kingwell E, Rieckmann P, Tremlett H, Neurologists UMC. The natural history of secondary progressive multiple sclerosis. *J Neurol Neurosurg Psychiatry*. 2010;81:1039-1043.
3   Lublin FD, Reingold SC. Defining the clinical course of multiple sclerosis: results of an international survey. National Multiple Sclerosis Society (USA) Advisory Committee on Clinical Trials of New Agents in Multiple Sclerosis. *Neurology*. 1996;46:907-911.
4   Lublin FD, Reingold SC, Cohen JA, et al. Defining the clinical course of multiple sclerosis: the 2013 revisions. *Neurology*. 2014;83:278-286.
5   Polman C, Reingold SC, Banwell, B., et al. Diagnostic criteria for multiple sclerosis: 2010 revisions to the McDonald Criteria. *Ann Neurol*. 2011;69:292-302.6.
6   Katz Sand I, Krieger S, Farrell C, Miller AE. Diagnostic uncertainty during the transition to secondary progressive multiple sclerosis. *Mult Scler*. 2014;20:1654-1657.
7   Bosma L, Kragt JJ, Polman CH, Uitdehaag BM. Walking speed, rather than Expanded Disability Status Scale, relates to long-term patient-reported impact in progressive MS. *Mult Scler*. 2013;19:326-333.
8   Bosma LV, Kragt JJ, Knol DL, Polman CH, Uitdehaag BM. Clinical scales in progressive MS: predicting long-term disability. *Mult Scler*. 2012;18:345-350.
9   Coleman CI, Sobieraj DM, Marinucci LN. Minimally important clinical difference of the Timed 25-Foot Walk Test: results from a randomized controlled trial in patients with multiple sclerosis. *Curr Med Res Opin*. 2012;28:49-56.
10 Hobart J, Blight AR, Goodman A, Lynn F, Putzki N. Timed 25-foot walk: direct evidence that improving 20% or greater is clinically meaningful in MS. *Neurology*. 2013;80:1509-1517.

11 Schwid SR, Goodman AD, McDermott MP, Bever CF, Cook SD. Quantitative functional measures in MS: what is a reliable change? *Neurology*. 2002;58:1294-1296.

12 Kragt JJ, van der Linden FA, Nielsen JM, Uitdehaag BM, Polman CH. Clinical impact of 20% worsening on Timed 25-foot Walk and 9-hole Peg Test in multiple sclerosis. *Mult Scler*. 2006;12:594-598.

13 van Winsen LM, Kragt JJ, Hoogervorst EL, Polman CH, Uitdehaag BM. Outcome measurement in multiple sclerosis: detection of clinically relevant improvement. *Mult Scler*. 2010;16:604-610.

14 Lassmann H, van Horssen J, Mahad D. Progressive multiple sclerosis: pathology and pathogenesis. *Nat Rev Neurol*. 2012;8:647-656.

15 Placebo-controlled multicentre randomised trial of interferon beta-1b in treatment of secondary progressive multiple sclerosis. European Study Group on interferon beta-1b in secondary progressive MS. *Lancet*. 1998;352:1491-1497.

16 Panitch H, Miller A, Paty D, Weinshenker B; North American Study Group on Interferon beta-1b in Secondary Progressive MS. Interferon beta-1b in secondary progressive MS: results from a 3-year controlled study. *Neurology*. 2004;63:1788-1795.

17 Kappos L, Weinshenker B, Pozzilli C, et al. Interferon beta-1b in secondary progressive MS: a combined analysis of the two trials. *Neurology*. 2004;63:1779-1787.

18 Cohen JA, Cutter GR, Fischer JS, Goodman AD, Heidenreich FR, Kooijmans MF, et al. Benefit of interferon beta-1a on MSFC progression in secondary progressive MS. *Neurology*. 2002;59:679-687.

19 Secondary Progressive Efficacy Clinical Trial of Recombinant Interferon-Beta-1a in MS (SPECTRIMS) study group. Randomized controlled trial of interferon- beta-1a in secondary progressive MS: clinical results. *Neurology*. 2001;56:1496-1504.

20 Andersen O, Elovaara I, Farkkila M, et al. Multicentre, randomised, double blind, placebo controlled, phase III study of weekly, low dose, subcutaneous interferon beta-1a in secondary progressive multiple sclerosis. *J Neurol Neurosurg Psychiatry*. 2004;75:706-710.

21 La Mantia L, Vacchi L, Di Pietrantonj C, et al. Interferon beta for secondary progressive multiple sclerosis. *Cochrane Database Syst Rev*. 2012;1:CD005181.

22 Confavreux C, Vukusic S, Moreau T, Adeleine P. Relapses and progression of disability in multiple sclerosis. *N Engl J Med*. 2000;343:1430-1438.

23 Paz Soldan MM, Novotna M, Abou Zeid N, et al. Relapses and disability accumulation in progressive multiple sclerosis. *Neurology*. 2015;84:81-88.

24 Martinelli Boneschi F, Vacchi L, Rovaris M, Capra R, Comi G. Mitoxantrone for multiple sclerosis. *Cochrane Database Syst Rev*. 2013;5:CD002127.

Walking disability in multiple sclerosis

Sarah Morrow

History

A 60-year-old woman was originally diagnosed with relapsing-remitting multiple sclerosis (RRMS) in 1972. Ten years ago, she began to notice a slow progression in her disease, specifically with her ambulation. Although she is currently mobilizing with the aid of a cane in her house, she has increasingly needed bilateral assistance; she uses walls or furniture to steady herself at home and often holds on to a companion when ambulating outside. She has fallen four times in the last few months and in each instance only had her cane to stabilize herself.

Examination

On examination, she was afebrile and in no distress. She was able to walk 30 meters with bilateral assistance before needing to rest. Visual acuity in the left eye was 20/50 and counting fingers in the right eye due to a previous severe optic neuritis. She had saccadic pursuit and nystagmus on lateral gaze bilaterally, but full extraocular movements. Her speech was mildly dysarthric. She had mild weakness in a pyramidal distribution in her right arm. In the lower extremities, she had 3/5 power in right leg with a foot drop, and mild pyramidal distribution weakness (4/5 to 4+/5) on the left. She had significantly increased tone in both legs. She had absent vibration sense to the level of the sternum on the right and to the coastal margin on the left. She had mild dysmetria on

© Springer International Publishing Switzerland 2017
P.S. Giacomini (ed.), *Case Studies in Multiple Sclerosis*,
DOI 10.1007/978-3-319-31190-6_11

finger-to-nose testing bilaterally. Her gait was spastic, wide-based, and ataxic. Her Expanded Disability Status Scale (EDSS) score was 6.5. On a Timed 25-Foot Walk (T25-FW) test, she completed her first attempt in 14.3 seconds and 12.0 seconds on the second attempt, both while using a walker.

Outcome

Following this evaluation, her physician prescribed fampridine sustained-release (SR) 10 mg every 12 hours. One month later, she called the clinic to state she felt better on this medication and wanted to continue. She was evaluated at a routine visit 3 months later and noted that since the addition of fampridine SR, she had an improvement in her stamina and fatigue, stating she could do more activities before feeling tired. She reported using her walker less often and felt more stable when using her cane. She still used her cane or walker when outside the home, as she was concerned about uneven ground, but was now able to use the cane less often in her house. She performed the T25-FW with her cane in 12.8 seconds on the first attempt and 11.7 seconds on the second attempt. She is now able to walk 100 meters with her cane and her EDSS is 6.0.

Discussion

Fampridine SR (chemical name: 4-aminopyridine) is an extended-release formulation of fampridine, a potassium channel blocker. Although it is not fully understood how fampridine SR exerts its therapeutic effect, the hypothesis is based on the fact that demyelinated axons do not effectively conduct action potentials, partly due to abnormal potassium currents that contribute to conduction failure by decreasing action potential duration and amplitude. Thus, potassium channel blockers, such as 4-aminopyridine, are thought to improve nerve impulse propagation by decreasing the leaking of current through these channels, enhancing action potential formation, and improving conduction by preventing conduction block [1,2].

Fampridine SR is indicated for the symptomatic improvement of walking in adult patients with multiple sclerosis (MS) with evidence of walking disability (EDSS 3.5/4.0–7.0).

Two Phase III placebo-controlled clinical trials demonstrated an improvement in ambulation, fatigue, and endurance in patients with MS given fampridine SR [3–6]. Compared to patients on placebo, significantly more patients with MS taking fampridine SR 10 mg twice daily increased walking speed on the T25-FW (34.8% vs. 8.3% and 42.9% vs. 9.3%) [7,8]. Approximately half of the study population had secondary progressive MS (SPMS) and, although this response was noted in all MS types, the SPMS group demonstrated a 39.7% improvement on the T25-FW [9]. In addition to improving walking speed, a recent randomized placebo-controlled study demonstrated that fampridine SR also improves both static and dynamic balance [10].

Importantly, these studies suggested there is a 'responder effect,' meaning subjects with MS who do respond to the medication may respond very well. A responder was defined as an increase in walking speed in those given fampridine, compared to placebo run-in, for at least three of four assessments during the trial [7]. Responders showed greater improvement in walking speed (25.2% vs. 4.7%) and subjective ratings of walking ability (change of –6.8 vs. 0.05) [7]. However, it was noted that responders could be identified as early as the first and second week after the initiation of treatment as there was a significant difference between responders and non-responders by this point in the study. After discontinuation of fampridine, T25-FW scores returned to baseline within a week. The most common adverse events noted were dizziness and insomnia (36% each), paresthesia (32%), asthenia (28%), nausea (28%), headache (24%), and tremor (24%) [11]. However, the majority of adverse events were transient in nature and only mild or moderate in severity. Urinary tract infections were also more commonly noted in the treatment group (12%) when compared to placebo (8%) [11].

Fampridine SR is excreted by the kidney and the elimination half-life is 5.2–6.5 hours [11]. Fampridine SR clearance is decreased in patients with renal impairment and, thus, use in patients with renal impairment is contraindicated. Due to renal excretion, there is the potential for interactions with other drugs that are renally excreted, specifically organic cation transporter inhibitors such as cimetidine and quinidine [11].

Seizures rarely occurred in placebo-controlled trials (fampridine SR 1/532 [0.19%] vs. placebo 1/249 [0.4%]), and this is a known risk of fampridine SR. There is a dose-dependent increase in risk of seizures at doses above the recommended dose. Thus, the recommended daily dose of 10 mg taken 12 hours apart should not be exceeded. Patients with a prior history or current presentation of seizure, or considered to be at high risk of seizure, should not start treatment with fampridine SR [11]. Careful consideration should be noted in patients on other medications known to lower seizure threshold and if a seizure occurs while on fampridine SR it should be discontinued immediately. Although there is no clear evidence that the use of fampridine SR in combination with other medications that lower seizure threshold, such as bupropion or metronidazole, will increase the risk of seizures, the addition of these medications in patients with MS using fampridine SR should be done cautiously. Finally, it should be emphasized with the patient that the two daily doses should be taken 12 hours apart and on an empty stomach.

The risk of seizures is also increased with renal impairment, due to reduced clearance of fampridine SR. Prior to starting treatment, renal function, specifically creatinine clearance, should be determined. Fampridine SR should not be started until the creatinine clearance is obtained and fits within the parameters set out by the appropriate federal health agency (eg, Health Canada or the US Food and Drug Administration). Due the renal route of clearance with fampridine SR, renal impairment can lead to increased risk of seizures due to increasing levels of fampridine SR in the serum.

Finally, there are published case reports of worsening of trigeminal neuralgia symptoms in patients with MS treated with fampridine SR. One retrospective case series noted that, out of five patients with MS and a history of trigeminal neuralgia, three had a worsening of facial pain with fampridine SR treatment [12].

Baseline assessment with an objective walking test such as the T25-FW should be done. The initial prescription should be for no more than 4 weeks, and assessment for improvement in walking should be carried out within that time frame, repeating the objective walking test performed at baseline, as well as subjective assessment of benefit from the patient.

For those at risk of renal impairment, routine monitoring for a change in renal function should be performed.

Clinical pearls

- Fampridine SR is indicated for use in patients with SPMS and an EDSS of 3.5–7.0. It has been shown in randomized placebo-controlled trials to improve walking speed, endurance, and balance.

- Fampridine SR is excreted by the kidney and a measure of creatinine clearance must be obtained prior to starting this medication. Monitoring for changes in creatinine clearance in high-risk patients is recommended. Caution is recommended when using other medications that are also renally excreted.

- Fampridine SR is contraindicated if there is a history of seizures; it is important to counsel the patient to take the medication 12 hours apart and not to exceed the recommended dose of 10 mg twice-daily, as increased serum levels increase the risk of seizures.

References

1   Shi R, Kelly TM, Blight AR. Conduction block in acute and chronic spinal cord injury: different dose-response characteristics for reversal by 4-aminopyridine. *Exp Neurol*. 1997;148:495-501.
2   Blight AR. Effect of 4-aminopyridine on axonal conduction-block in chronic spinal cord injury. *Brain Res Bull*. 1989;22:47-52.
3   van Diemen HA, Polman CH, van Dongen TM, et al. The effect of 4-aminopyridine on clinical signs in multiple sclerosis: a randomized, placebo-controlled, double-blind, cross-over study. *Ann Neurol*. 1992;32:123-130.
4   Bever CT, Jr., Young D, Anderson PA, et al. The effects of 4-aminopyridine in multiple sclerosis patients: results of a randomized, placebo-controlled, double-blind, concentration-controlled, crossover trial. *Neurology*. 1994;44:1054-1059.
5   Schwid SR, Petrie MD, McDermott MP, Tierney DS, Mason DH, Goodman AD. Quantitative assessment of sustained-release 4-aminopyridine for symptomatic treatment of multiple sclerosis. *Neurology*. 1997;48:817-821.
6   Stefoski D, Davis FA, Fitzsimmons WE, Luskin SS, Rush J, Parkhurst GW. 4-aminopyridine in multiple sclerosis: prolonged administration. *Neurology*. 1991;41:1344-1348.
7   Goodman AD, Brown TR, Krupp LB, et al. Sustained-release oral fampridine in multiple sclerosis: a randomised, double-blind, controlled trial. *Lancet*. 2009;373:732-738.
8   Goodman AD, Cohen JA, Cross A, et al. Fampridine-SR in multiple sclerosis: a randomized, double-blind, placebo-controlled, dose-ranging study. *Mult Scler*. 2007;13:357-368.
9   Brown T, Schapiro R, Goodman AD; MS-F202, MS-F203 and MS-F204 study groups. Response to treatment with prolonged-release fampridine tablets in patients with multiple sclerosis is independent of demographic, clinical, and patient-reported characteristics. Presented at: European Committee for Treatment and Research in Multiple Sclerosis (ECTRIMS); October 13-16, 2010; Gothenburg, Sweden.

10   Hupperts R, Lycke J, Short C, et al. Prolonged-release fampridine and walking and balance in MS: randomised controlled MOBILE trial. *Mult Scler*. 2015.

11   Biogen Idec Canada. Fampyra Product Monograph. 2012. Last updated November 26, 2014. www.biogen.ca/content/dam/corporate/en_CA/pdfs/products/ FAMPRYA/28November2014-Fampyra-PM-E.pdf. Accessed April 6, 2016.

12   Birnbaum G, Iverson J. Dalfampridine may activate latent trigeminal neuralgia in patients with multiple sclerosis. *Neurology*. 2014;83:1610-1612.

Cognitive impairment

Sarah Morrow

History

A 52-year-old man with a 24-year history of multiple sclerosis (MS) presented for his annual visit with his neurologist. His last relapse was 11 years prior and since that time he noted a slow worsening of his MS symptoms and has been formally diagnosed with secondary progressive (SPMS) for 7 years. He has never been on any disease-modifying therapy (DMT). He is otherwise healthy but does smoke a pack of cigarettes per day and drinks approximately eight beers per week. His main symptoms had been fatigue, which responds well to modafinil, and bladder urgency. However, his main complaint during this visit pertained to his memory.

On further questioning, he stated that, in retrospect, he suspects his memory symptoms began around the time of his diagnosis with relapsing-remitting (RRMS), but they have clearly worsened in the last year. Recently, he noticed he had difficulty maintaining his train of thought; he often gets distracted and has trouble finishing his sentences. He also noticed that unless he writes something down immediately, he will quickly forget it. He does not think anyone at work has noticed this trouble with his memory, but they are aware of his MS diagnosis and have always made accommodation for him. He has not received any reprimands at work.

His wife reports she has noticed his short-term memory problems over the last year as well. She reported that in the past, he would occasionally forget when she asked him to do something, but now he rarely remembers anything she asks if she doesn't remind him multiple times. At first, he

© Springer International Publishing Switzerland 2017
P.S. Giacomini (ed.), *Case Studies in Multiple Sclerosis*,
DOI 10.1007/978-3-319-31190-6_12

attributed these lapses to his fatigue, saying he was often too tired to do the requested task, but then did admit that he had not remembered to do the tasks she requested. Over the past year, both he and his wife started writing all important dates and events on a calendar and he started programming multiple reminders on his phone.

He also noted difficulty following multiple conversations during social gatherings or if multiple people are talking to him at the same time. He has also noticed that he has been becoming more 'moody'. He reported becoming easily frustrated and that he has difficulty, as he describes it, 'coming out of it'. He does not have a history of depression, anxiety, or any other psychiatric diagnoses.

Examination

In the clinic, he appeared well groomed and dressed appropriately. He was able to give his history without difficulty and was alert and oriented. On self-reported measures, there was evidence of moderate generalized fatigue, as well as mild anxiety and depressive symptoms. On objective testing, he performed in the moderate-to-severe impairment range on information processing speed tests, and was moderately impaired on measures of immediate and delayed recall.

Outcome

This patient is suffering from cognitive impairment (CI) associated with MS. Significant difficuties with short-term memory and concentration are characteristic of MS-related CI.

Discussion

Although disease duration and physical disability do not predict the presence of CI, there is a relationship with disease type and time since diagnosis [1,2]. CI is known to be more frequent and more severe in progressive types of MS than in RRMS [1,3,4]. CI is been found in up to 60% of patients with SPMS [5].

Unlike Alzheimer's dementia and other cortical dementias characterized by aphasia, apraxia, and agnosia [6], CI presentation in MS is more similar to subcortical dementias affecting information processing speed, memory, and executive function, manifesting as a profound slowing of cognition (bradyphrenia) [6,7]. Additionally, psychiatric and personality changes are common, specifically cognitive inflexibility, apathy, irritability, and mood disorders such as depression and anxiety [3,8].

CI in MS most frequently involves information processing speed, new learning, and memory [3,5], as well as verbal fluency, visual spatial abilities, and executive function [9,10]. CI in MS is slowly progressive and shows little evidence of improvement once established [11–13]. More recently, it has been demonstrated that acute inflammatory lesions (relapses) can affect cognition [14,15]. Thus, it is likely that both inflammation and neurodegeneration contribute to CI in MS.

The onset of CI in MS can be subtle and is frequently missed during routine clinical assessments. Patients with MS who are cognitively impaired are more likely to report loss of self-esteem, participate in fewer social activities, and have higher rates of divorce [16,17]. Both cross-sectional studies and longitudinal studies indicate that CI is the strongest predictor of patients with MS reducing work responsibilities or leaving the work force [18–20].

There are multiple factors that can either exacerbate or cause CI to occur in a pattern that can mimic MS. Other potential causes of CI should always be considered, specifically medications such as pregabalin, opiates, and medications with anticholinergic effects [21–24]. Generalized fatigue, a common symptom in SPMS, with a lifetime prevalence of 75–95% [25,26], is also known to be associated with subjectively reported poor cognitive performance. Yet, studies examining the relationship between fatigue and objective cognitive performance have not noted an objective worsening of CI with worsening fatigue, with the exception of performance on the Symbol Digit Modalities Test (SDMT) [27].

Anxiety and depression are also quite common in MS, with lifetime prevalence rates of 35% for anxiety and between 25–50% for depression [28–30]. Anxiety is well known to be associated with subjectively reported poor cognitive performance [31]. Finally, depression, especially when in the moderate-to-severe range, can worsen performance on objective cognitive tests, and can also lead to overestimation of the degree of CI when self-evaluating cognitive function [32,33].

Screening for cognitive impairment

It is recommended that screening for CI be performed every 2 or 3 years for patients with MS [34]. Identification of CI in a standard clinical assessment can be difficult, as the presentation and symptoms can be subtle in onset. Recently, a screening battery called the Brief International Cognitive Assessment for MS (BiCAMS), composed of a measure of processing speed and two measures of immediate recall, was proposed as a short screening tool to be used in a clinic setting [35]. There is also a computerized cognitive test battery specifically made for use with the MS population [36]. The SDMT, a measure of information processing speed, has also been proposed as a screening tool [5,37]. Studies show the SDMT maintains validity with repeated testing, and worsening on the SDMT is associated with clinically relevant changes such as employment [19,38]. It takes only 5 minutes to administer and score.

However, all these tests require an additional person to administer the test. This is not always feasible in a clinical setting, especially in a busy clinical practice. The Multiple Sclerosis Neuropsychological Screening Questionnaire (MSNQ) was developed as a self-report and informant version subjective questionnaire which, similar to our semi-structured interview tool, used clinically relevant questions when screening for the presence of CI [33]. The self-report tool, although quite useful, was found to be significantly confounded by depression or mood symptoms. By contrast, the informant-report was found to be sensitive and specific [39], although the use of an informant-only tool is not always practical. Thus, although no one screening test can be definitively recommended, the use of one test consistently (to allow for monitoring of change over time) will help enable the clinician to identify those patients with SPMS who require more comprehensive testing, such as a full neuropsychological assessment.

Clinical pearls

- CI is common in SPMS and usually presents with subtle findings that are insidiously progressive over time and have a significant impact on quality of life.

- When evaluating a patient with SPMS for CI, other factors such as medications, mood disorders, and fatigue must also be considered and evaluated.
- Screening for CI in SPMS should occur at least every 2 or 3 years; although no one test has been found to be the ideal screening test, one screening test or battery should be used consistently in order to monitor for change over time.

References

1   Achiron A, Chapman J, Magalashvili D, et al. Modeling of cognitive impairment by disease duration in multiple sclerosis: a cross-sectional study. *PLoS One*. 2013;8:e71058.

2   Amato MP, Zipoli V, Goretti B, et al. Benign multiple sclerosis: cognitive, psychological and social aspects in a clinical cohort. *J Neurol*. 2006;253:1054-1059.

3   Rao SM, Leo GJ, Bernardin L, Unverzagt F. Cognitive dysfunction in multiple sclerosis. I. Frequency, patterns, and prediction. *Neurology*. 1991;41:685-691.

4   Achiron A, Polliack M, Rao SM, et al. Cognitive patterns and progression in multiple sclerosis: construction and validation of percentile curves. *J Neurol Neurosurg Psychiatry*. 2005;76:744-749.

5   Benedict RH, Cookfair D, Gavett R, et al. Validity of the minimal assessment of cognitive function in multiple sclerosis (MACFIMS). *J Int Neuropsychol Soc.*. 2006;12:549-558.

6   Cummings JL. Subcortical dementia. Neuropsychology, neuropsychiatry, and pathophysiology. *Br J Psychiatry*. 1986;149:682-697.

7   Turner MA, Moran NF, Kopelman MD. Subcortical dementia. *Br J Psychiatry*. 2002;180:148-151.

8   Aarsland D, Karlsen K. Neuropsychiatric aspects of Parkinson's disease. *Curr Psychiatry Rep*. 1999;1:61-68.

9   Chiaravalloti ND, DeLuca J. Cognitive impairment in multiple sclerosis. *Lancet Neurol*. 2008;7:1139-1151.

10   Benedict RH, Fischer JS, Archibald CJ, et al. Minimal neuropsychological assessment of MS patients: a consensus approach. *Clin Neuropsychol*. 2002;16:381-397.

11   Duque B, Sepulcre J, Bejarano B, Samaranch L, Pastor P, Villoslada P. Memory decline evolves independently of disease activity in MS. *Mult Scler*. 2008;14:947-953.

12   Kujala P, Portin R, Ruutiainen J. The progress of cognitive decline in multiple sclerosis. A controlled 3-year follow-up. *Brain*. 1997;120 (Pt 2):289-297.

13   Amato MP, Portaccio E, Goretti B, et al. Relevance of cognitive deterioration in early relapsing-remitting MS: a 3-year follow-up study. *Mult Scler*. 2010;16:1474-1482.

14   Morrow SA, Jurgensen S, Forrestal F, Munchauer FE, Benedict RH. Effects of acute relapses on neuropsychological status in multiple sclerosis patients. *J Neurol*. 2011;258:1603-1608.

15   Benedict RH, Morrow S, Rodgers J, et al. Characterizing cognitive function during relapse in multiple sclerosis. *Mult Scler*. 2014;20:1745-52.

16   Rao SM, Leo GJ, Ellington L, Nauertz T, Bernardin L, Unverzagt F. Cognitive dysfunction in multiple sclerosis. II. Impact on employment and social functioning. *Neurology*. 1991;41:692-696.

17   Hakim EA, Bakheit AM, Bryant TN, Roberts MW, McIntosh-Michaelis SA, Spackman AJ, et al. The social impact of multiple sclerosis--a study of 305 patients and their relatives. *Disabil Rehabil*. 2000;22:288-293.

18   Ruet A, Deloire M, Hamel D, Ouallet JC, Petry K, Brochet B. Cognitive impairment, health-related quality of life and vocational status at early stages of multiple sclerosis: a 7-year longitudinal study. *J Neurol*. 2013;260:776-784.

19 Morrow SA, Drake A, Zivadinov R, Munschauer F, Weinstock-Guttman B, Benedict RH. Predicting loss of employment over three years in multiple sclerosis: clinically meaningful cognitive decline. *Clin Neuropsychol*. 2010;24:1131-1145.

20 Flensner G, Landtblom AM, Soderhamn O, Ek AC. Work capacity and health-related quality of life among individuals with multiple sclerosis reduced by fatigue: a cross-sectional study. *BMC Public Health*. 2013;13:224.

21 Katz IR, Sands LP, Bilker W, DiFilippo S, Boyce A, D'Angelo K. Identification of medications that cause cognitive impairment in older people: the case of oxybutynin chloride. *J Am Geriatr Soc*. 1998;46:8-13.

22 Low LF, Anstey KJ, Sachdev P. Use of medications with anticholinergic properties and cognitive function in a young-old community sample. *Int J Geriatr Psychiatry*. 2009;24:578-584.

23 Salinsky M, Storzbach D, Munoz S. Cognitive effects of pregabalin in healthy volunteers: a double-blind, placebo-controlled trial. *Neurology*. 2010;74:755-761.

24 Oken BS, Flegal K, Zajdel D, et al. Cognition and fatigue in multiple sclerosis: Potential effects of medications with central nervous system activity. *J Rehabil Res Dev*. 2006;43:83-90.

25 Lerdal A, Celius EG, Krupp L, Dahl AA. A prospective study of patterns of fatigue in multiple sclerosis. *Eur J Neurol*. 2007;14:1338-1343.

26 Freal JE, Kraft GH, Coryell JK. Symptomatic fatigue in multiple sclerosis. *Arch Phys Med Rehabil*. 1984;65:135-138.

27 Morrow SA, Weinstock-Guttman B, Munschauer FE, Hojnacki D, Benedict RH. Subjective fatigue is not associated with cognitive impairment in multiple sclerosis: cross-sectional and longitudinal analysis. *Mult Scler*. 2009;15:998-1005.

28 Korostil M, Feinstein A. Anxiety disorders and their clinical correlates in multiple sclerosis patients. *Mult Scler*. 2007;13:67-72.

29 Minden SL, Schiffer RB. Affective disorders in multiple sclerosis. Review and recommendations for clinical research. *Arch Neurol*. 1990;47:98-104.

30 Siegert RJ, Abernethy DA. Depression in multiple sclerosis: a review. *J Neurol Neurosurg Psychiatry*. 2005;76:469-475.

31 Akbar N, Honarmand K, Feinstein A. Self-assessment of cognition in Multiple Sclerosis: the role of personality and anxiety. *Cogn Behav Neurol*. 2011;24:115-121.

32 Demaree HA, Gaudino E, DeLuca J. The relationship between depressive symptoms and cognitive dysfunction in multiple sclerosis. *Cogn Neuropsychiatry*. 2003;8:161-171.

33 Benedict RH, Munschauer F, Linn R, et al. Screening for multiple sclerosis cognitive impairment using a self-administered 15-item questionnaire. *Mult Scler*. 2003;9:95-101.

34 Freedman MS, Selchen D, Arnold DL, et al. Treatment optimization in MS: Canadian MS Working Group updated recommendations. *Can J Neurol Sci*. 2013;40:307-323.

35 Langdon DW, Amato MP, Boringa J, et al. Recommendations for a Brief International Cognitive Assessment for Multiple Sclerosis (BICAMS). *Mult Scler*. 2012;18:891-898.

36 Lapshin H, Lanctot KL, O'Connor P, Feinstein A. Assessing the validity of a computer-generated cognitive screening instrument for patients with multiple sclerosis. *Mult Scler*. 2013;19:1905-1912.

37 Van Schependom J, D'Hooghe M B, Cleynhens K, et al. The Symbol Digit Modalities Test as sentinel test for cognitive impairment in multiple sclerosis. *Eur J Neurol*. 2014;21:1219-1225.

38 Morrow S, O'Connor P, Polman C, et al. Evaluation of the symbol digit modalities test (SDMT) and MS neuropsychological screening questionnaire (MSNQ) in natalizumab-treated MS patients over 48 weeks. *Mult Scler*. 2010;16:1385-1392.

39 Benedict RH, Cox D, Thompson LL, Foley F, Weinstock-Guttman B, Munschauer F. Reliable screening for neuropsychological impairment in multiple sclerosis. *Mult Scler*. 2004;10:675-678.

Pediatric Multiple Sclerosis and Related Disorders

Acute disseminated encephalomyelitis

Sunita Venkateswaran

History

The mother of a 6-year-old girl noticed that her daughter was 'walking funny' when she picked her up from school. That evening, the child did not want to eat her dinner and fell asleep earlier than usual. She did not complain of any other symptoms. The next morning, the child was unable to get out of bed on her own and was quite unsteady. She had an episode of nocturnal enuresis after being dry overnight for 2 years. Her speech was dysarthric and she had difficulty brushing her teeth. She was not interested in eating and was very irritable. She was afebrile and did not have any rhinorrhea, vomiting, or diarrhea. She had not had any sick contacts.

Her past medical history was unremarkable. She was born at term after an uncomplicated pregnancy to a 25-year-old gravida 1 mother (first child). There were no neonatal complications and her development to date was appropriate. She is currently in grade 1 and an average student. She has not had any medical admissions or surgeries. Her family history was not significant for developmental, neurological, or metabolic disorders.

She was taken to the local emergency room by her parents. Her height, weight, and head circumference were in the 75th percentile. She was very irritable and was challenging to examine. Her parents repeatedly stated that this behavior was unlike their daughter.

© Springer International Publishing Switzerland 2017
P.S. Giacomini (ed.), *Case Studies in Multiple Sclerosis*,
DOI 10.1007/978-3-319-31190-6_13

99

Examination

Her vital signs were stable and within normal limits. She was afebrile, did not have meningismus, and had no rashes or joint swelling. There was no lymphadenopathy. Cardiac, respiratory, and abdominal exams were normal.

Upon neurological examination, there was a right relative afferent pupillary defect. Her fundi appeared normal. She had full extraocular movements. Facial movements were symmetrical. Her gag response was intact. Her speech was dysarthric and nonsensical.

She was unable to sit up on her own and exhibited truncal ataxia. Muscle tone was normal. Power was difficult to assess, but appeared to be within normal limits. Reflexes were brisk in the lower extremities. Plantar responses were both upgoing. Sensation could not be reliably assessed. Her abdominal reflexes were intact. She exhibited bilateral dysmetria when trying to reach for objects. She could not walk.

Investigations

An MRI of the brain and spinal cord showed asymmetrical, poorly demarcated T2-weighted hyperintense lesions involving the subcortical and periventricular white matter, as well as the deep gray matter (basal ganglia and thalami) (Figure 13.1). Cerebrospinal fluid (CSF) analysis showed a lymphocytosis (66 white blood cells [WBC]/mm^3) with minimally elevated protein and no oligoclonal bands. However, all infectious tests and cultures were negative on the CSF.

Outcome

After imaging and investigations excluded all other potential causes, she was diagnosed with acute disseminated encephalomyelitis (ADEM). Treatment with intravenous steroids was then started and she began to recover within a few days of treatment initiation.

Discussion

ADEM is a presumed inflammatory condition of the central nervous system that may involve both the brain and the spinal cord. The diagnosis is made based on clinical presentation, supported by MRI and CSF findings,

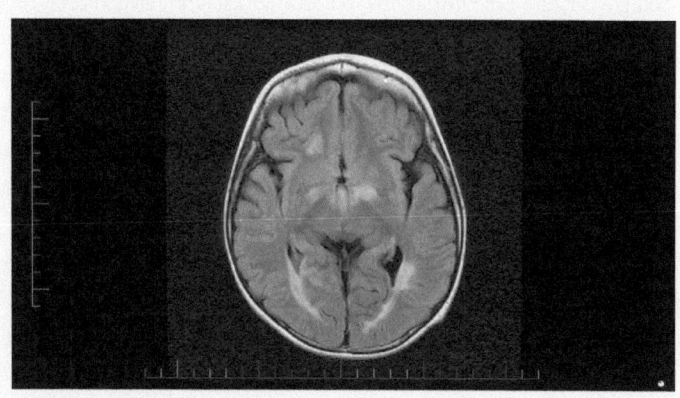

Figure 13.1 Axial T2 weighted FLAIR MRI demonstrating asymmetrical, poorly demarcated lesions involving the subcortical and periventricular white matter and the deep gray matter (basal ganglia and thalami).

and the exclusion of other conditions. The patient may present with a multifocal neurological presentation: symptoms and signs attributable to multiple areas of CNS involvement with encephalopathy [1]. Children are usually young, but it can present at any age. Symptoms can include pyramidal tract involvement (60–95%), ataxia (18–65%), optic neuritis (7–23%), acute hemiplegia (76%), cranial nerve involvement (22–45%), dysarthria (5–21%), and seizures (13–35%) [2]. Peripheral nervous system involvement is rarely reported. The child is encephalopathic (eg, major behavioral change, change in level of arousal) that is beyond what is in keeping with the child being unwell. Typically, the child may have been ill with a non-specific upper respiratory tract infection or may have been vaccinated in the month prior to presentation. The nadir of symptoms usually occurs within 2–5 days of onset. Children can become sick enough to require ventilator support in extreme cases and, therefore, they should be monitored diligently upon presentation.

Diagnosis
The diagnosis of ADEM is one of exclusion [3]. There are no biomarkers that can confirm the diagnosis. Care must be taken to exclude other treatable causes of CNS inflammation including CNS infections, both viral

and bacterial. Some etiologies to consider include bacterial meningitis, viral encephalitis due to Epstein–Barr virus, herpes viruses, enteroviruses, tuberculosis, and mycoplasma. In an immunocompromised population, HIV, cytomegalovirus, and fungal infections should be tested for and excluded. In certain regions, West Nile virus and arboviruses may mimic an ADEM presentation. Other autoantibody syndromes (eg, neuromyeltis optica, anti-N-methyl-D-aspartate [NMDA] receptor encephalitis, anti-myelin oligodendrocyte glycoprotein antibody syndrome) are continually being further characterized and should be tested for based on clinical presentation. Rheumatologic illnesses such as systemic lupus erythematosus, sarcoidosis, Behçet's disease, and CNS vasculitis may also mimic ADEM. Tumors and hematological conditions (eg, lymphoma, hemophagocytic lymphohistiocytosis) should also be taken into consideration, especially prior to starting treatments such as corticosteroids. Neurometabolic and neurogenetic conditions such as mitochondrial disorders, organic acidopathies, and leukodystrophies can also present acutely in the context of an illness or precipitant; imaging can further assist in determining the likelihood of these conditions.

ADEM, although typically monophasic, can also be the first presentation of multiple sclerosis (MS) or neuromyelitis optica spectrum disorder (NMOSD). 'Red flags' to warrant consideration of a diagnosis other than ADEM include pre-existing developmental delay or regression, epilepsy, multisystemic involvement, peripheral neuropathy (as it is rarely seen in ADEM), and atypical MRI findings. Investigations for ADEM are outlined in Table 13.1.

It is most important that MRI and CSF studies are performed acutely, ideally prior to initiation of treatment, as subsequent investigations are guided by these results. CSF typically shows pleocytosis, typically not more than 100 WBC/mm^3. Opening pressure and biochemistry should be within normal limits. Oligoclonal banding can be present, but occurs in less than 30% of cases. MRI typically demonstrates both subcortical and deep grey matter abnormalities that are widespread, asymmetrical, and poorly demarcated; they may or may not enhance. Both the spinal cord and optic nerves should be evaluated with appropriate MRI sequences, as

Investigations to consider	
Test	**Measurement**
Bloodwork	Complete blood count (CBC) and differential
	Liver enzymes
	Renal function
	Inflammatory markers:
	• antinuclear antibody (ANA)
	• double-stranded DNA
	• erythrocyte sedimentation rate (ESR)
	• C-reactive protein (CRP)
	• C3/C4
	• antiphospholipid antibodies (APLA)
	• anticardiolipin antibody (ACLA)
	Vitamin B_{12}, 25(OH) Vitamin D
	Ferritin
	Triglycerides
	Lactate
	Angiotensin-converting enzyme (ACE)
	Antibody studies:
	• neuromyelitis optica (NMO)
	• N-methyl-D-aspartate receptor (NMDAR)
	• thyroid peroxidase antibodies (TPO)
	• myelin oligodendrocyte glycoprotein (MOG)
	Bacterial and viral studies *
	DNA banking
Throat and nasal swab	Mycoplasma polymerase chain reaction (PCR)
	Routine virus*
Stool sample	Enterovirus
Imaging	MRI brain ± orbits ± spine with gadolinium, MRA, MRV, MRS as indicated
	Chest X-ray (if suspecting hemophagocytic lymphohistiocytosis or sarcoidosis)
CSF studies	Culture and sensitivity (C&S), cell count, protein, glucose, oligoclonal banding
	Cytology
	Viral studies:
	• West Nile
	• Epstein–Barr
	• Enterovirus
	• Varicella zoster
	• Cytomegalovirus
	• Human T-lymphotropic virus 1 (HTLV-1)
	• HIV
	Fungal cultures
	NMO immunoglobulin G (IgG)
	ACE

Table 13.1 Investigations to consider in a child presenting with an acute demyelinating syndrome (continues overleaf).

Investigations to consider	
Test	**Measurement**
Ancillary testing	Optical coherence tomography (OCT)
	Evoked potentials (VEP, SSEP, ABER)
	Electroencephalogram (EEG)
Consultations	Ophthalmology
	Urology
	Psychiatry
	Social work
	Neuropsychology
	Physiotherapy

Table 13.1 Investigations to consider in a child presenting with an acute demyelinating syndrome (continued). *Serum viral studies may include Epstein-Barr virus, serology, herpes simplex virus 1, human herpesvirus 6, Lyme antibodies, measles, mumps, rubella, influenza, varicella zoster, cytomegalovirus, parvovirus B19, venereal disease research laboratory (VDRL), West Nile, and arboviruses. Serum bacterial studies may include *Bartonella henselae*, *Mycoplasma*, and *Mycobacterium tuberculosis*. ABER, auditory brain stem evoked reponse; MRA, magnetic resonance angiography; MRS, magnetic resonance spectroscopy; MRV, magnetic resonance venography; SSEP, somatosensory evoked potential; VEP, visually evoked potential.

these lesions can be subclinical. Hemorrhage can signify a serious subtype of ADEM known as acute hemorrhagic leukoencephalomyelitis (AHEM).

Clinical improvement typically occurs before the MRI improves. Most children will have complete resolution of their MRI lesions over a 3-month period, and the lack of resolution or the appearance of new lesions at this time should prompt further investigations. Ancillary investigations should include evoked potentials, especially visual evoked potentials as optic neuritis in this population can be easily missed clinically.

As soon as other treatable causes such as infections have been ruled out, the standard treatment is intravenous methylprednisolone [4]. The dosing is 20–30 mg/kg/day for 5 days to a maximum dose of 1 g/day. If the patient is suspected to have a CNS lymphoma, is immunocompromised, or may have tuberculosis or a fungal infection, then steroids should not be given until these conditions are ruled out. Children can start showing some improvement after 3 days of treatment. In some cases, intravenous (IV) methylprednisolone may need to be repeated. Intravenous immunoglobulin (IVIg), although not an established therapy, can be given in situations where patients have worsened or not improved with IV steroid treatment.

In cases where there has been a severe decline in neurological function leading to intensive care monitoring, or minimal response to steroid and IVIg therapy, it may be appropriate to use plasma exchange [4]. There is no clear role for oral steroid tapering following IV steroids, and this is a decision made on a case-by-case basis.

According to studies based on the International Pediatric Multiple Sclerosis Study Group (IPMSSG) consensus definition [1], most cases of ADEM remain monophasic; therefore, the term 'recurrent ADEM' is no longer used.

Multiphasic ADEM is also infrequent. This entity consists of two distinct episodes of ADEM at least 3 months apart, affecting new or previously involved areas of the CNS based on clinical and MRI findings. MS and other chronic demyelinating conditions, including NMOSD, should be considered when there is a second demyelinating event 3 months after the initial ADEM event, if it does not meet the definition of ADEM (eg, without encephalopathy), with new MRI findings meeting the criteria for dissemination in space. Most children with monophasic ADEM recover completely but a small proportion, especially those under the age of 5, may exhibit cognitive or behavioral sequelae.

Clinical pearls

- ADEM is a clinical diagnosis with supportive investigations. Children must have both multifocal neurological signs and encephalopathy.
- ADEM has a wide differential diagnosis in children. Treatable conditions such as meningitis, encephalitis and auto-antibody syndromes should be considered and ruled out before a diagnosis can be made.
- ADEM can involve the optic nerves and spinal cord and therefore imaging of the brain and spinal cord, as well as evoked potentials, are advised.
- Imaging in ADEM is not symmetrical in nature. If symmetrical lesions are noted, metabolic and genetic conditions such as organic

acidurias, mitochondrial diseases, leukodystrophies, and other rare entities must be considered.

- Although most cases of ADEM are monophasic, a small proportion of children can have a relapse. Therefore, children with ADEM should be followed for clinical or radiological relapses. Some of these children with relapses may subsequently be given a diagnosis of MS or another chronic CNS inflammatory condition.

References

1   Krupp LB, Tardieu M, Amato MP, et al; International Pediatric Multiple Sclerosis Study Group. International Pediatric Multiple Sclerosis Study Group criteria for pediatric multiple sclerosis and immune-mediated central nervous system demyelinating disorders: revisions to the 2007 definitions. *Mult Scler.* 2013;19:1261-1267.

2   Tenembaum S. Acute disseminated encephalomyelitis. *Handb Clin Neurol.* 2013;112:1253-1262.

3   Rostasy K, Bajer-Kornek B, Venkateswaran S, Hemingway C, Tardieu M. Differential diagnosis and evaluation in pediatric demyelinating disorders. *Neurology.* In press.

4   Pohl D, Tenembaum S. Treatment of acute disseminated encephalomyelitis. *Curr Treat Options Neurol.* 2012;14:264-275.

Pediatric multiple sclerosis

Sunita Venkateswaran

History

A 13-year-old previously healthy girl complained of a two-day history of double vision. She has a family history of aneurysms on her paternal side, but did not have a headache and denied any recent head trauma or infectious symptoms. She did not have joint pain, ulcers, or rashes. She has no pets (specifically cats). She lives in a downtown apartment and has not been outside the city in the last several months.

Examination

On examination, she has horizontal diplopia on rightward gaze and full abduction of the right eye with some nystagmus. The left eye can only adduct to midline. Horizontal gaze to the left is full without nystagmus or diplopia. Vertical gaze is intact. There is no pain with extraocular movements. Pupils are equal and reactive to light. Visual acuity is normal. Examination of the fundi is normal. The rest of the cranial nerve exam is intact. There are no other abnormalities on neurological examination.

Investigations

She underwent an MRI scan (Figure 14.1). A lumbar puncture revealed normal white blood cell count and biochemistry, but was positive for oligoclonal bands. Her symptoms resolved over a 4-week period without any treatment.

© Springer International Publishing Switzerland 2017

P.S. Giacomini (ed.), *Case Studies in Multiple Sclerosis*,

DOI 10.1007/978-3-319-31190-6_14

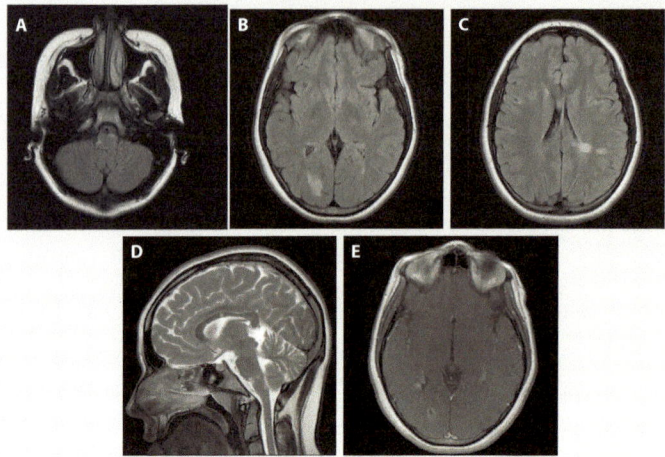

Figure 14.1 A 13-year-old girl with internuclear ophthalmoplegia. Axial FLAIR images demonstrating hyperintense lesions in (**A**) brainstem, (**B** and **C**) periventricular region, and (**C**) juxtacortical. (**D**) Sagittal T2-weighted image demonstrating intracallosal 'Dawson's fingers' and lesions in the pontomedullary junction. (**E**) T1 contrast enhancement of a juxtacortical lesion.

Outcome

One year later, while on a trip to the Caribbean, she developed numbness of her right leg and had difficulty walking. Upon her return home, she underwent a second MRI, showing two new lesions (when compared to the previous scan). She was given a diagnosis of multiple sclerosis (MS) after further investigations excluded potential mimics.

Discussion

This teenager's initial presentation is consistent with intranuclear ophthalmoplegia (INO). The top differential diagnosis for an INO in any age group is an acute demyelinating event, although vascular and infectious causes of a brainstem syndrome must be ruled out with imaging and a lumbar puncture. The presence of positive oligoclonal bands, with no evidence of an infection or rheumatological disease on cerebrospinal fluid (CSF) and serum studies, and imaging demonstrating discrete lesions in typical locations seen in a demyelinating syndrome, is consistent with a clinically isolated syndrome (CIS).

However, this patient could have also been diagnosed with MS on the basis of her first episode, as long as certain imaging criteria are present. According to the 2010 McDonald MS diagnostic criteria [1], should a child have a first demyelinating attack that is typical of a CIS and the MRI shows evidence of dissemination in time and space, then the child can be diagnosed with MS at that time. In this particular case, the patient's MRI demonstrated an asymptomatic gadolinium-enhancing lesion that was not responsible for her current symptoms, demonstrating dissemination in time. She also had lesions in the periventricular and juxtacortical white matter, in addition to the lesions in the brainstem, thereby meeting the criteria for dissemination in space.

One caveat to the 2010 McDonald criteria is the situation where the child presents with acute disseminated encephalomyelitis (ADEM) [1]. ADEM is not considered a typical CIS presentation and, therefore, even if the MRI lesions meet the criteria for dissemination in space and time, a second attack must occur. At this point, if the attack is typical of a demyelinating event in MS, and there is further imaging evidence supporting the diagnosis, plus exclusion of other causes, a diagnosis of MS can be made. Although the current McDonald criteria does not exclude children younger than 10 years of age, care must be taken to do a thorough work-up for younger children to ensure they do not have a disorder that mimics the symptoms of MS.

Children can have similar CIS presentations to adults including optic neuritis, transverse myelitis, and other monofocal or multifocal demyelinating episodes [2]. Risk factors for having a subsequent demyelinating event confirming the diagnosis of MS (when the first event does not meet the diagnostic criteria) include more than one T2 hyperintense lesion on MRI, positive oligoclonal bands, and an age of CIS onset of ≥12 years [3].

The work-up for a child presenting with CIS is similar to the work-up for a child presenting with ADEM (see Table 13.1). 'Red flags' for neurological illnesses other than a CIS include encephalopathy, parental consanguinity, prior developmental delay, a progressive course, peripheral nerve involvement, seizures, and prominent psychiatric symptoms [4].

Imaging that demonstrates symmetrical changes should prompt evaluation of metabolic and genetic conditions. Children may not complain of visual loss and, therefore, evoked potentials and ophthalmological examination should be done on every child to rule out optic neuritis. An MRI should also include a T1 fat-saturated coronal image to evaluate the optic nerves. Spinal cord MRI should be strongly considered in all children. Younger children may not have bowel and bladder control at baseline, and so spinal cord imaging may reveal an otherwise subclinical lesion. Serum studies should evaluate and exclude infectious and rheumatological conditions. Lumbar puncture should include, at a minimum, biochemistry, cell count, viral and bacterial studies, and oligoclonal bands. In children, many autoantibody conditions can mimic CIS and, therefore, antibodies to aquaporin-4/neuromyelitis optica, N-methyl-D-aspartate (NMDA) receptor, and myelin oligodendrocyte glycoprotein may also be considered. If a metabolic condition is being considered, CSF lactate and amino acids should also be collected. Tumefactive lesions should prompt cytology studies.

Treatment

For an acute relapse, if causing moderate-to-severe neurological deficits, as with adults, IV methylprednisolone (30 mg/kg/day for 5 days, maximum of 1 g) or high-dose oral prednisone can be prescribed for 5 days [5].

Disease-modifying therapies can be used as with adults but this is off-label use. The medications most commonly used in children include interferon and glatiramer acetate. While none of these medications have been formally evaluated in children in prospective clinical trials, retrospective studies have demonstrated their safety [5]. Contraceptive options must be discussed with any adolescent starting a disease-modifying therapy.

The newer medications used in adults, including natalizumab, fingolimod, alemtuzumab, and dimethyl fumarate, have not yet been evaluated in pediatric MS clinical trials. These newer medications should not be used outside of a clinical trial, as per the International Pediatric MS Study Group recommendations [6]. Natalizumab has been used in aggressive cases of pediatric MS at highly specialized pediatric MS centers, with very close monitoring. The long-term consequences of using these therapies in children are still unknown and areas of particular concern include later impact on fertility and the risk of secondary malignancies.

Several pediatric MS clinical trials are ongoing and details can be found on www.clinicaltrials.gov.

Disease course in pediatric patients

Previous studies have looked at the natural history of children with pediatric MS. The majority of children (98%) have a relapsing-remitting course. Children also tend to recover well from their early relapses. The second MS-defining attack typically occurs within 2 years of the CIS event. If there is ongoing progression or incomplete recovery after successive attacks, the diagnosis should be reconsidered. Although children tend to appear 'well' early in the course of their illness and typically take 10 years longer than adults to enter secondary progression, they usually enter the secondary progressive phase of MS in their fourth decade of life [7].

Furthermore, although children and teenagers with MS may seem physically well in between attacks, recent studies underscore that the cognitive impact of MS in children is profound. Brain growth is already on a different trajectory at the time of diagnosis, with brain size being smaller in children with MS when compared to healthy controls [8,9]. This signifies that the impact of MS pathology is already being felt years prior to clinical presentation. Verbal skills appear relatively preserved, masking the areas of difficulty, including visuospatial learning [10]. Children with MS tend to fatigue more easily than peers and modifications to learning styles and scheduling for both physical and academic activities may be necessary. Neuropsychological testing should be performed at baseline in every child diagnosed with MS so that appropriate educational resources can be put in place as promptly as possible.

Clinical pearls

- Based on the 2010 McDonald MS diagnostic criteria, MS can be diagnosed in children at the time of the first demyelinating event, as long as the first event is consistent with a CIS (not ADEM), MRI demonstrates both dissemination in time and space, and other potential diagnoses have been excluded.

- There is evidence that MS pathology is already underway in children before the initial demyelinating event, as brain growth is affected early on.
- Aggressive cases should be referred to a pediatric MS center for therapeutic guidance. Newer therapies should only be given in the context of a pediatric MS clinical trial.
- Children with MS suffer from neurocognitive consequences and should be evaluated early in the course of their illness and have appropriate measures in place to optimize their education.

References

1   Polman CH, Reingold SC, Banwell B, et al. Diagnostic criteria for multiple sclerosis: 2010 revisions to the McDonald criteria. *Ann Neurol*. 2011;69:292-302.

2   Waldman A, Ghezzi A, Bar-Or A, Mikaeloff Y, Tardieu M, Banwell B. Multiple sclerosis in children: an update on clinical diagnosis, therapeutic strategies and research. *Lancet Neurol*. 2014;13:936-948.

3   Banwell B, Bar-Or A, Arnold DL, et al. Clinical, environmental, and genetic determinants of multiple sclerosis in children with acute demyelination: a prospective national cohort study. *Lancet Neurol*. 2011;10:436-445.

4   Venkateswaran S, Banwell B. Pediatric multiple sclerosis. *Neurologist*. 2010;16:92-105.

5   Narula S, Hopkins SE, Banwell B. Treatment of pediatric multiple sclerosis. *Curr Treat Options Neurol*. 2015;17:336.

6   Chitnis T, Tardieu M, Amato MP, et al. International Pediatric MS Study Group Clinical Trials Summit: meeting report. *Neurology*. 2013;80:1161-1168.

7   Renoux C, Vukusic S, Mikaeloff Y, et al; Adult Neurology Departments KIDMUS Study Group. Natural history of multiple sclerosis with childhood onset. *N Engl J Med*. 2007;356:2603-2613.

8   Kerbrat A, Aubert-Broche B, Fonov V, et al. Reduced head and brain size for age and disproportionately smaller thalami in child-onset MS. *Neurology*. 2012;78:194-201.

9   Aubert-Broche B, Fonov V, et al; Canadian Pediatric Demyelinating Disease Network. Onset of multiple sclerosis before adulthood leads to failure of age-expected brain growth. *Neurology*. 2014;83:2140-2146.

10 Amato MP, Goretti B, Ghezzi A, et al; MS Study Group of the Italian Neurological Society. Neuropsychological features in childhood and juvenile multiple sclerosis: five year follow-up. *Neurology*. 2014;83:1432-1438.

Pediatric multiple sclerosis mimics

Sunita Venkateswaran

History

A 3-year-old boy is admitted to a hospital after a two-day history of a mild upper respiratory tract illness. He presented with confusion, irritability, and slurred speech. As the day progressed, he developed difficulty swallowing.

Examination

He was afebrile with vital signs in the normal range. He was uncooperative and displayed very little extraocular or facial movements. His gag reflex was minimal. His tone was increased in all four limbs and he appeared rigid, with intermittent dystonic posturing of his hands and feet. Reflexes were brisk and plantar responses were both upgoing. He was intubated and ventilated due to the inability to protect his airway.

Investigations

An emergent CT scan was performed. It appeared normal with no signs of infarction, increased intracranial pressure, or bleeding. A lumbar puncture was performed and the spinal fluid analysis did not reveal any signs of an infection. An MRI performed later that same day showed symmetrical involvement of the striatum (Figure 15.1).

Outcome

This patient's clinical presentation is consistent with a subacute encephalopathy. His clinical symptoms, signs, and imaging are all unusual for

© Springer International Publishing Switzerland 2017
P.S. Giacomini (ed.), *Case Studies in Multiple Sclerosis*,
DOI 10.1007/978-3-319-31190-6_15

multiple sclerosis (MS), and this presentation has a broad differential diagnosis and warrants a thorough series of investigations.

Discussion

This young child is presenting with a subacute encephalopathy and after ruling out meningoencephalitis, the clinician must next consider other treatable disorders. This child did not appear to be in subclinical status epilepticus; but if any doubt, an electroencephalogram should be

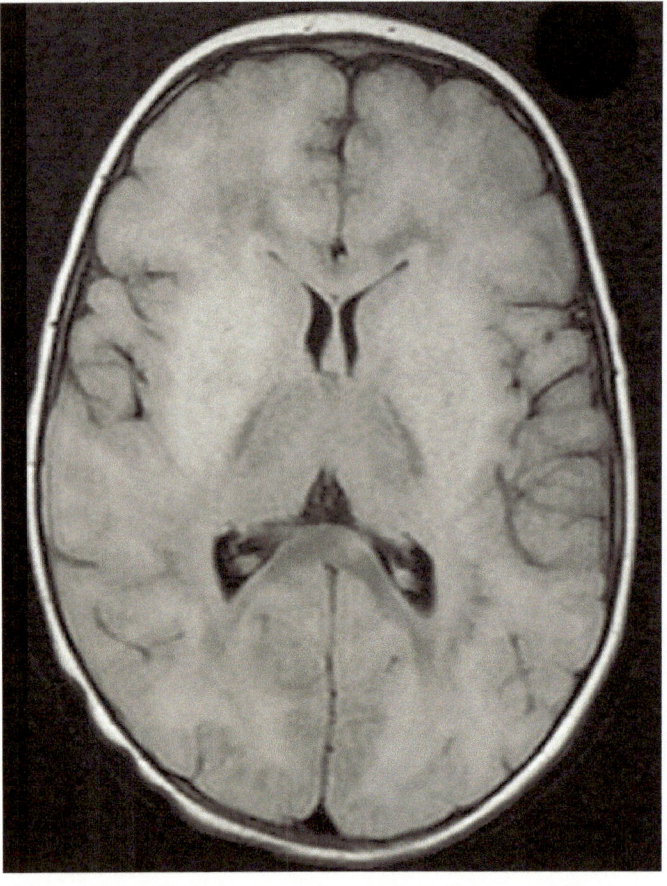

Figure 15.1 Axial T2 FLAIR MRI demonstrating symmetric involvement of the basal ganglia, thalami, and subcortical white matter regions.

performed urgently, or intravenous (IV) abortive antiepileptic therapy may be given empirically to ensure that this is not part of the presentation.

Initial imaging with CT ruled out trauma, large infarction, and a hemorrhage. Acute demyelinating encephalomyelitis (ADEM) may present in this manner but many disorders, especially metabolic disorders, may also mimic ADEM [1]. In particular, mitochondrial disorders, amino acidopathies, organic acidurias, urea cycle defects, and toxic encephalopathies are all part of the differential diagnosis. Metabolic disorders may even be acutely precipitated by non-specific illnesses and present with a rapid evolution.

An MRI demonstrating symmetrical grey/white matter changes should immediately alert the clinician to evaluate for infectious, neurometabolic, and genetic disorders, especially those that are treatable [2]. Conditions that primarily involve the basal ganglia include Leigh syndrome, biotin-thiamine responsive basal ganglia disease (BTRBG), Wernicke's encephalopathy, osmotic demyelination, and toxins (methanol and cyanide preferentially affecting the putamen, carbon monoxide preferentially affecting the globus pallidus). Encephalitides such as Japanese B encephalitis also have a predilection for the basal ganglia. These conditions have a predilection for the basal ganglia, as they are highly metabolic structures and particularly vulnerable to metabolic derangements. When thalamic involvement is prominent, acute necrotizing encephalopathy (a genetic cause of acute encephalopathy) should also be included in the differential diagnosis [3].

In addition to broad-spectrum antibiotics and possibly antivirals, initial management should include controlling any increased intracranial pressure, fever, and seizures. Furthermore, therapies should be considered for treatable metabolic conditions such as amino acidopathies, organic acidurias, urea cycle defects, and Wilson disease. In this particular case, based on imaging findings and clinical presentation, biotin and thiamine were administered presuming BTRBG [4]. This is an autosomal recessive condition presenting with seizures, encephalopathy, and involvement of both pyramidal and extrapyramidal systems (spasticity, hyperreflexia, prominent dystonia, and rigidity), typically triggered by a non-specific illness [4]. This disease typically presents in childhood subacutely, although there are cases with preceding progressive dystonia and developmental delays followed by an episode. Administering biotin and thiamine can dramatically improve the symptoms within days. The sooner therapy is administered, the better the outcome.

This disease is caused by mutations in the *SLC19A3* gene, which encodes a thiamine transporter [5]. Family members identified with this mutation should also be started on biotin and thiamine, even if asymptomatic. Stresses such as fever, trauma, and surgery can trigger a relapse and, therefore, these children should have regular follow-ups, with anticipatory guidance in place to avoid and control these stresses as much as possible.

Clinical pearls

- Symmetrical abnormalities on MRI should alert the clinician to consider metabolic and genetic disorders.
- Treatable causes of demyelination should be considered in every child presenting with acute encephalopathy.
- If a genetic or metabolic cause of recurrent demyelinating disease is identified, appropriate anticipatory guidance and close follow-up should be in place to prevent future exacerbations or relapses.

References

1   Rostasy K, Bajer-Kornek B, Venkateswaran S, Hemingway C, Tardieu M. Differential diagnosis and evaluation in pediatric demyelinating disorders. *Neurology*. In press.

2   Zuccoli G, Yannes MP, Nardone R, Bailey A, Goldstein A. Bilateral symmetrical basal ganglia and thalamic lesions in children: an update. *Neuroradiology*. 2015;57:973-989.

3   Neilson DE, Adams MD, Orr CM, et al. Infection triggered acute necrotizing encephalopathy caused by mutations in a component of the nuclear pore, RANBP2. *Am J Hum Genet*. 2009;84:44-51.

4   Tabarki B, Al-Shafi S, Al-Shahwan S, et al. Biotin-responsive basal ganglia disease revisited: clinical, radiologic, and genetic findings. *Neurology*. 2013;80:261-267.

5   Zeng WQ, Al-Yamani E, Acierno JS Jr, et al. Biotin-responsive basal ganglia disease maps to 2q36.3 and is due to mutations in SLC19A3. *Am J Hum Genet*. 2005;77:16-26.

Pregnancy and Multiple Sclerosis

Prenatal planning in multiple sclerosis

Matthew R. Lincoln and Jiwon Oh

History

A 24-year-old, right-handed woman presented with a three-day history of worsening left monocular visual loss. She initially noted an 'oily smudge' over her central visual field while using her computer at work. Bright colors were less vibrant. Symptoms progressed over the next 2 days to visual loss involving most of the left monocular visual field. For the past day, she noted left retro-orbital pain, particularly at the extremes of eye movement. When she covered the left eye, vision with the right eye was normal. There were no other neurological symptoms and no history of previous transient neurological symptoms. Her past medical history was unremarkable and she took no regular medications. There was no family history of neurologic or autoimmune disease.

Examination

Vital signs and general medical examination were unremarkable. Cognition was normal. On cranial nerve examination, visual acuities were 20/20-1 in the right eye and 20/80 in the left. She correctly identified 17/17 Ishihara plates with the right eye and 10/17 with the left. There was a left relative afferent pupillary defect (grade 2+). Both optic discs appeared normal. Extraocular movements were normal and there was no evidence of internuclear ophthalmoplegia. The remainder of

© Springer International Publishing Switzerland 2017
P.S. Giacomini (ed.), *Case Studies in Multiple Sclerosis*,
DOI 10.1007/978-3-319-31190-6_16

the cranial nerves were normal. Motor and sensory examinations were unremarkable. There was no ataxia. Gait and tandem gait were normal.

Investigations

The clinical findings were highly suggestive of optic neuritis affecting the left eye. An MRI scan of the brain was requested, and revealed a few small T2 hyperintensities in the periventricular and juxtacortical white matter consistent with demyelination. A single lesion in the right frontal white matter enhanced after gadolinium contrast administration.

Outcome

A diagnosis of relapsing-remitting multiple sclerosis (RRMS) was made in concordance with the 2010 McDonald criteria [1]. Her symptoms improved completely over 2 weeks following a 5-day course of high-dose methylprednisolone.

She returned to clinic a month later for follow up and disease-modifying therapy was suggested, but the patient expressed concern about her future childbearing. Although she was not planning a pregnancy in the near future, she had heard from one of her friends that MS is genetic and that her children would be at risk. She was also concerned about potential birth defects and the effects of disease-modifying therapy on childbearing and the health of her future children.

Discussion

As MS typically affects women of childbearing age, this is a common clinical scenario in the MS clinic. Through the mid-20th century, women with MS were advised to avoid pregnancy out of concern that it would increase disease activity. Recommendations began to change after publication of the Pregnancy in Multiple Sclerosis (PRIMS) study [2]; this prospective study of 269 pregnancies in patients with MS revealed no net effect of pregnancy on disease activity over the study period, including pregnancy and the first year postpartum.

In fact, immune tolerance is enhanced in pregnancy, as the maternal immune system adapts to the presence of the foreign placental unit. Concordant with this model, the rate of relapse in the PRIMS study declined by about 70% in the third trimester compared to a pre-pregnancy baseline; this was balanced by a similar increase in the first 3 months postpartum, before the relapse rate returned to baseline [2]. Alterations in disease activity may be related to physiologic immune modulation that occurs with pregnancy.

The long-term data that are available also suggest that there is no definite negative impact of pregnancy on MS progression. Analysis of a large survey of patients with MS revealed a reduced risk of reaching Expanded Disability Status Scale (EDSS) score of 6.0 (unilateral assistance required to walk 100 meters) among patients with at least two pregnancies, compared to nulliparous women [3]. In contrast, a retrospective population-based, case-control study involving 305 patients with clinically isolated syndrome or early MS suggested that the use of hormonal contraceptives for at least 3 months in the 3 years prior to symptom onset increased disease risk [4]. These results are preliminary and the available data do not permit definitive recommendations on the use of hormonal contraception.

MS itself has no impact on fertility or on obstetrical outcomes. The risk of birth defect or miscarriage is not increased. Obstetrical risk is not increased. Contrary to previous orthodoxy, epidural anesthesia does not seem to increase disease activity [2,5].

For the fetus, the risk of developing MS is increased, but this risk remains low. A large population-based study of genetic risk demonstrated that first-degree relatives have a 3–5% age-adjusted risk of developing MS; this is compared to a lifetime prevalence in the general population of 0.2% [6]. Though this risk is increased, it remains small overall.

Though animal studies did not reveal adverse fetal outcomes, glatiramer acetate is classified by the Food and Drug Administration (FDA) as category B (Table 16.1) due to the absence of controlled human studies. Extensive experience with incidental glatiramer acetate exposure during pregnancy, however, revealed no evidence for increased congenital anomalies, low birth weight, preterm delivery, or spontaneous abortion [7–9]. Glatiramer acetate may be used safely up to 1 month before attempting conception and some neurologists may even treat patients with this agent throughout pregnancy, although this is not advised.

Category A

Adequate and well-controlled studies in pregnant women have failed to demonstrate a risk to the fetus in the first trimester of pregnancy (and there is no evidence of a risk in later trimesters).

Category B

Animal reproduction studies have failed to demonstrate a risk to the fetus and there are no adequate and well-controlled studies in pregnant women.

Category C

Animal reproduction studies have shown an adverse effect on the fetus and there are no adequate and well-controlled studies in humans. The benefits from the use of the drug in pregnant women may be acceptable despite its potential risks.

Category D

There is positive evidence of human fetal risk based on adverse reaction data from investigational or marketing experience or studies in humans, but the potential benefits from the use of the drug in pregnant women may be acceptable despite its potential risks.

Category X

Studies in animals or humans have demonstrated fetal abnormalities or if there is positive evidence of fetal risk based on adverse reaction reports from investigational or marketing experience, or both, and the risk of the use of the drug in a pregnant woman clearly outweighs any possible benefit.

Table 16.1 Food and Drug Administration (FDA) pregnancy categories. Reproduced with permission from FDA [10] ©FDA.

Interferons are classified FDA category C (Table 16.1), as studies in monkeys revealed an abortifacient effect at high doses [8]. Long-term experience with interferon use in humans has revealed no association with teratogenicity, spontaneous abortion, or low birth weight (<2500 g) [7,8]. However, though studies are inconclusive, there may be an association with preterm delivery, shorter mean birth length, and lower mean birth weight [7]. These agents have been used safely up to 1 month prior to attempting conception. Experience with the newer agents is still limited, but a longer washout period is generally recommended.

Clinical pearls

- Pregnancy is possible in MS and the disease itself has no impact on fertility, the rate of birth defects, or potential obstetrical complications.
- Pregnancy is a state of relative immune tolerance. The relapse rate declines in the third trimester, only to rebound by 3 months post-partum. Overall, there is no definite long-term negative impact of pregnancy on MS disease activity.

- The risk of MS in the offspring of an affected parent is increased in comparison to the general population risk, but remains low.
- Though none of the disease-modifying therapies in clinical use have been licensed for use during pregnancy, several therapies may be used safely prior to conception with an adequate washout period.

References

1 Polman CH, Reingold SC, Banwell B, et al. Diagnostic criteria for multiple sclerosis: 2010 revisions to the McDonald criteria. *Ann Neurol*. 2011;69292-692302.

2 Confavreux C, Hutchinson M, Hours MM, Cortinovis-Tourniaire P, Moreau T. Rate of pregnancy-related relapse in multiple sclerosis. Pregnancy in Multiple Sclerosis Group. *N Engl J Med*. 1998;339:285-291.

3 D'hooghe MB, Haentjens P, Nagels G, D'Hooghe T, De Keyser J. Menarche, oral contraceptives, pregnancy and progression of disability in relapsing onset and progressive onset multiple sclerosis. *J Neurol*. 2012;259:855-861.

4 Hellwig K, Chen L, Langer-Gould A. Hormonal contraceptives and multiple sclerosis susceptibility (S34.003). *Neurology*. 2014;82:S34.003.

5 Pastò L, Portaccio E, Ghezzi A, et al. Epidural analgesia and cesarean delivery in multiple sclerosis post-partum relapses: the Italian cohort study. *BMC Neurol*. 2012;12:165.

6 Sadovnick AD, Baird PA, Ward RH. Multiple sclerosis: updated risks for relatives. *Am J Med Genet*. 1988;29:533-541.

7 Lu E, Wang BW, Guimond C, Synnes A, Sadovnick D, Tremlett H. Disease-modifying drugs for multiple sclerosis in pregnancy: a systematic review. *Neurology*. 2012;79:1130-1135.

8 Houtchens MK, Kolb C. M. Multiple sclerosis and pregnancy: therapeutic considerations. *J Neurol*. 2013;260:1202-1214.

9 Cree BA. Update on reproductive safety of current and emerging disease-modifying therapies for multiple sclerosis. *Mult Scler*. 2013;19:835-843.

10 Food and Drug Administration (FDA). Content and format of labeling for human prescription drug and biological products. Requirements for pregnancy and lactation labeling. *Federal Register*. 2008;73:30831-30868.

Multiple sclerosis therapies and pregnancy

Matthew R. Lincoln and Jiwon Oh

History

A 24-year-old patient (see Case 16) with relapsing-remitting multiple sclerosis (RRMS) returned 6 months after diagnosis with sub-acute diplopia. She described difficulty moving her eyes to the right and horizontal, binocular diplopia, maximal in leftward gaze. There were no other neurological symptoms. Examination revealed conjugate horizontal gaze palsy to the right and limited adduction of the right eye, constituting the 'one-and-a-half syndrome.' A repeat MRI scan revealed a new lesion in the right pons affecting the region of the abducens nucleus and the ipsilateral medial longitudinal fasciculus. There was no enhancement. The overall burden of lesions on MRI was otherwise stable, and the enhancing right frontal lesion previously seen was less prominent.

She was treated with a 5-day course of high-dose intravenous (IV) methylprednisolone and made a full recovery over several weeks. Following this second attack, she elected to begin disease-modifying therapy (DMT) with dimethyl fumarate. She remained stable and free of relapses for the next 2 years. At that point, she began to trip on the left leg when she walked. This became more frequent over the next 3 days and she noticed that the left leg was weaker than the right. She felt less able to control the left foot and worried it would give out under her. There were no sensory symptoms and her bowel and bladder function were normal.

© Springer International Publishing Switzerland 2017
P.S. Giacomini (ed.), *Case Studies in Multiple Sclerosis*,
DOI 10.1007/978-3-319-31190-6_17

Examination

Her exam revealed a mild degree of spasticity in the left leg. There was also a mild degree of weakness in the left leg (4+/5), especially involving hip flexion, knee flexion, and ankle dorsiflexion. Reflexes were more brisk in the left leg compared to the right and the left plantar response was extensor. Sensory examination was normal. Her symptoms were felt to reflect an acute partial myelitis.

Investigations

MRI scan of the spinal cord revealed a small T2 hyperintense lesion involving the left corticospinal tract at T8. She again made a full recovery over several weeks following a course of IV methylprednisolone. When she returned to clinic a month later, she felt well and her neurological examination was normal. Unfortunately, repeat MRI of her brain revealed multiple new T2 hyperintense lesions in the periventricular and juxtacortical white matter. Several of these enhanced with gadolinium contrast. Given the clinical and radiological evidence of disease activity, she elected to discontinue dimethyl fumarate and begin treatment with teriflunomide.

Outcome

One year later, she returned for a follow-up visit feeling well. She was promoted at work and recently purchased a new home. She and her partner were contemplating pregnancy within the next year. She recalled previous advice that she would have to discontinue teriflunomide several months prior to conception and this concerned her. She wanted to know what would happen if she experienced a relapse during pregnancy.

Discussion

This scenario illustrates the importance of pre-pregnancy planning for patients with multiple sclerosis. None of the current DMTs for multiple sclerosis (MS) have been approved for use in pregnancy and some of the newer agents are associated with teratogenicity. Though there are no evidence-based guidelines for the use of these agents around pregnancy, a washout period of variable length is generally advised. As washout could leave patients relatively unprotected from recurrent inflammation, neurologists generally recommend that patients attempt pregnancy once disease activity is relatively controlled, particularly for patients with very active disease.

Decades of experience with glatiramer acetate and the interferons have produced ample data on their use in and around pregnancy. While similar data are sparse for the newer agents, pregnancy registries have now accrued data from hundreds of pregnancies for many of the newer agents (Table 17.1). The newer agents each have specific toxicities that must be considered in the context of pregnancy.

Experience with dimethyl fumarate in pregnancy is limited to 27 live births from 45 pregnancies that occurred in clinical trials (Table 17.2) [1]. There were three spontaneous and ten therapeutic abortions in the same study. Though there have been no birth defects recorded, a single elective termination occurred following the identification of anomalies on ultrasound. Animal studies have also shown embryotoxicity and delayed ossification at high doses [2]. Given these potential risks, dimethyl fumarate has been classified by the Food and Drug Administration (FDA) as pregnancy category C (Table 17.1) and it is advisable to discontinue dimethyl fumarate 1–3 months prior to attempted conception.

Fingolimod exposure has been documented in 66 pregnancies (Table 17.1), from which there have been 28 live births; in the same cohort, there were 9 spontaneous and 24 therapeutic abortions [3]. Among the 28 live births, there was a single case of unilateral posteromedial bowing of the tibia and a single case of acrania. In addition, elective abortions were performed in four cases where anomalies were detected on ultrasound; these consisted of a single case of Tetralogy of Fallot (a congenital heart defect) and a single case each of ectopic pregnancy, intrauterine death, and failure of fetal development. Animal studies have also demonstrated teratogenicity [4]. Given these data, fingolimod has been placed in FDA pregnancy category C (Table 17.1) and it seems prudent to discontinue fingolimod at least 2 months prior to conception.

Clinical trials of teriflunomide have documented 70 pregnancies with exposure to teriflunomide and these resulted in 26 live births (Table 17.2). There were 29 therapeutic and 13 spontaneous abortions but no congenital anomalies [5]. Animal studies, however, demonstrated embryotoxicity

| | Oral therapies | | | Infusion therapies | |
	Teriflunomide	Dimethyl fumarate	Fingolimod	Alemtuzumab	Natalizumab
Patient exposure	6800 patient-years in clinical trials	2898 patients in clinical trials	7702 patient-years in clinical trials	1486 patients in clinical trials	375 patients (prospective study)
Data cut-off	October 18, 2013	June 30, 2014	October 31, 2011	October 17, 2013	May 23, 2012
Pregnancies (n)	70	45	66	139	362
Live births (n)	26	27	28	67	314
Spontaneous abortions (n [%])*	13 (18.6)	3 (6.7)	9 (13.6)	24 (17.2)	34 (9.4)
Birth defects (n [%])	0	0	2 (3.0)	0	28 (7.7)
Elective terminations (n [%])	29 (41.4)	10 (22.2)	24 (36.4)	14 (10.0)	13 (3.5)
Teratogenicity in animal studies	Yes	No	Yes	No	No
Pregnancy section in product monograph	Must be excluded**	Not recommended	Not recommended	Not recommended	–
Notes	None of the therapeutic abortions were due to structural defects or malformations	One elective termination was in the setting of abnormalities detected on ultrasound after at least 1 month off dimethyl fumarate	Therapeutic abortions were performed for one case each of Tetralogy of Fallot, spontaneous intrauterine death, and failure of fetal development	Therapeutic abortions were performed for one case each of anembryonic pregnancy and fetal defects identified on ultrasound	Includes patients who received natalizumab for the treatment of Crohn's disease

Table 17.1 Pregnancy outcomes with new disease-modifying therapies. *Normal range of spontaneous abortions in women without MS: 17–22%. **Pregnancy must be excluded before the start of treatment.

and teratogenicity. Given these risks, teriflunomide is classified as FDA pregnancy category X (Table 17.1) and a negative pregnancy test should be obtained prior to commencing therapy. Patients should use reliable contraception while using the medication. A washout period (Table 17.2) is required and serum levels should be <0.02 mg/L prior to attempting conception. As teriflunomide is secreted in semen and may be absorbed trans-vaginally, men are recommended not to father a child while on the drug [6].

A total of 375 pregnant patients exposed to natalizumab have been prospectively ascertained by the Tysabri® Pregnancy Exposure Registry and outcomes are available on 362 pregnancies [7]; there have been 314 live births, 1 stillbirth, 34 spontaneous, and 13 therapeutic abortions. Though teratogenicity was not observed in animal studies, natalizumab produced fetal hematologic effects and reduced offspring survival when administered at high dose [8]. To date, there have been a total of 28 birth defects in 26 pregnancies. Natalizumab has been classified as pregnancy category C by the FDA (Table 17.1).

Alemtuzumab is classified by the FDA as pregnancy category C (Table 17.1). Animal studies show reduced fetal viability when the drug was administered in high doses during gestation [9]. Human experience in pregnancy is limited to 139 pregnancies resulting in 67 live births (Table 17.2).

Agent	FDA pregnancy category	Minimum washout period
Glatiramer acetate	B	Discontinue at least 1 month prior to attempting conception
Interferon beta	C	Discontinue at least 1 month prior to attempting conception
Dimethyl fumarate	C	Discontinue 1–3 months prior to attempting conception
Fingolimod	C	Discontinue at least 2 months prior to attempting conception
Teriflunomide	X	Accelerated elimination prior to attempting conception and confirm serum levels <0.02 mg/L
Natalizumab	C	Discontinue 1–3 months prior to attempting conception
Alemtuzumab	C	Discontinue at least 4 months prior to attempting conception

Table 17.2 Recommended minimum wash-out periods for multiple sclerosis disease-modifying therapies. These are recommendations based on available evidence and expert opinion, but all clinical decisions should only be undertaken after thorough discussion of risk and benefit between patient and doctor.

There were 24 spontaneous and 14 therapeutic abortions [10]. Therapeutic abortion was performed for one anembryonic pregnancy and another case where fetal defects were identified on an ultrasound. There was a single case of thyrotoxic crisis in an infant born to a mother who developed Grave's disease during pregnancy [10].

Treatment of symptomatic relapses in pregnancy should be carefully considered. Steroids should be avoided wherever possible in the first trimester as these may cross the placenta and increase the risk of cleft palate and lower birth weight. Where required, prednisone, prednisolone, and methylprednisolone should be favored over betamethasone and dexamethasone, as the former agents are metabolized to inactive forms by the placenta. In contrast, betamethasone and dexamethasone cross the placenta unmetabolized, which could result in detrimental effects to the developing fetus.

Clinical pearls

- Clinical experience with the new generation of DMTs in MS is limited, but a longer washout period prior to conception is generally advised.
- Symptomatic relapses in pregnancy may be treated with pulse doses of steroid. Prednisone, prednisolone, and methylprednisolone are favored over dexamethasone and betamethasone.

References

1   Gold R, Theodore Phillips J, Havrdova E, et al. P839 Delayed-release dimethyl fumarate and pregnancy: preclinical studies and pregnancy outcomes from clinical trials and postmarketing experience. *Neurol Ther*. 2015;1-12.

2   Wei QR, Runrong G, Xiangdong S. Studies on teratogenicity of dimethyl fumarate. *J Hyg Res*. 1990;19:28-31.

3   Karlsson G, Francis G, Koren G, et al. Pregnancy outcomes in the clinical development program of fingolimod in multiple sclerosis. *Neurology*. 2014;82:674-680.

4   Novartis Pharmaceuticals Corporation. Gilenya (fingolimod) prescribing information (2010). Revised August 2015. www.accessdata.fda.gov/drugsatfda_docs/label/2015/022527s019lbl.pdf. Accessed April 6, 2016.

5   Kieseier BC, Benamor M, Truffinet P, Henson LJ. Pregnancy outcomes for female patients and partners of male patients in the teriflunomide clinical development program. Presented at: ACTRIMS-ECTRIMS; September 12, 2014; Boston, Massachusetts, USA. Poster P846.

6   Genzyme Corporation. Aubagio (teriflunomide) prescribing information. Revised October 2014a. http://products.sanofi.us/aubagio/aubagio.pdf. Accessed April 6, 2016.

7   Cristiano L, Friend S, Bozic C, Bloomgren G. Evaluation of pregnancy outcomes from the TYSABRI (Natalizumab) pregnancy exposure registry. *Neurology*. 2013;80(Meeting Abstracts 1):P02.127.

8   Biogen Idec Inc. Tysabri (natalizumab) prescribing information. Revised May 2015. www.tysabri.com/prescribingInfo. Accessed April 6, 2016.

9   Genzyme Corporation. Lemtrada (alemtuzumab) prescribing information. Revised November 2014. http://products.sanofi.us/lemtrada/lemtrada.pdf. Accessed April 6, 2016.

10   McCombe P, Achiron A, Brinar B, et al. Pregnancy outcomes in the alemtuzumab multiple sclerosis clinical development program. Presented at: ACTRIMS-ECTRIMS; September 12, 2014; Boston, Massachusetts, USA. Poster P842.

Postpartum issues with multiple sclerosis

Matthew R. Lincoln and Jiwon Oh

History

A patient with relapsing-remitting multiple sclerosis (RRMS) elected to pursue pregnancy (see Case 16 and 17). As she was currently prescribed teriflunomide, her medication needed to be halted and eliminated from the bloodstream, as it is contraindicated in pregnancy. As teriflunomide is eliminated slowly from the plasma, an accelerated elimination procedure is required [1]. Without accelerated elimination, an average of 8 months is required to reach the recommended preconceptual plasma level of less than 0.02 mg/L; in some patients, this may take up to 2 years. There are two recommended procedures for accelerated elimination of teriflunomide [2]. Under the first, cholestyramine is administered in a dose of 8 g every 8 hours for 11 days; if this is not well tolerated, a dose of 4 g three times a day may be used. An alternate regimen consists of 50 g of oral activated charcoal powder given every 12 hours for 11 days. After completing accelerated elimination with cholestyramine, the patient's serum teriflunomide levels were confirmed to be <0.02 mg/L. Contraception was discontinued and she conceived 4 months later.

Outcome

The pregnancy itself was uncomplicated and free of clinical relapse. A spontaneous vaginal delivery was successful under epidural anesthesia. She returned to the clinic for a follow-up. She has been breastfeeding

© Springer International Publishing Switzerland 2017   133
P.S. Giacomini (ed.), *Case Studies in Multiple Sclerosis*,
DOI 10.1007/978-3-319-31190-6_18

and would like to continue to do so, but is concerned about postpartum relapse. She asked if there are therapeutic agents that can be used safely while breastfeeding.

Discussion

Postpartum relapse is a significant concern for many patients with MS. The Pregnancy and Multiple Sclerosis (PRIMS) study demonstrated an increase in relapse rate in the first 3 months postpartum [1] and subsequent studies have suggested that this risk may be mitigated by exclusive breastfeeding, but the results are inconsistent [3–5]. Additionally, although the PRIMS study demonstrated the safety of breastfeeding in MS [1,6], concerns about secretion of disease-modifying therapies (DMTs) in breast milk remain and, accordingly, none of the available DMTs for MS are approved for use while breastfeeding.

Excretion of glatiramer acetate or interferon beta through breast milk is not clearly established [7], though oral absorption of the intact peptide is likely insignificant [8]. Nevertheless, use of these agents while breastfeeding is still not generally recommended. Fingolimod, teriflunomide, and dimethyl fumarate are secreted in breast milk; therefore, use of these agents while breastfeeding is not recommended. Similarly, infusion therapies are not recommended.

In the absence of evidence-based guidelines, clinical judgment and patient preference with regards to duration of breastfeeding plays an important role in the decision to resume DMT postpartum. In individuals who had very active disease pre-pregnancy, it may be advisable for these patients to resume DMT shortly after delivery, as the postpartum relapse risk tends to be proportional to the pre-pregnancy relapse rate [1]. As the available therapies take weeks to months to reach full therapeutic effect, some neurologists advocate using intravenous immunoglobulin as a therapeutic 'bridge,' though studies have been inconsistent [9–11]. As with treatment during pregnancy, the decision to resume DMT while breastfeeding should be made after careful consideration of all the risks and benefits, patient preference, and the patient's specific risk profile.

Clinical pearls

- Breastfeeding is safe in MS and exclusive breastfeeding may potentially mitigate the postpartum increase in relapse rate.
- Most of the available DMTs are secreted in breast milk and should not be used while breastfeeding.
- The timing of resuming DMT postpartum is an individual decision and a number of factors, including patient preference and risk of postpartum relapse, must be taken into account.

References

1 Vukusic S, Hutchinson M, Hours M, et al. Pregnancy and multiple sclerosis (the PRIMS study): clinical predictors of post-partum relapse. *Brain*. 2004;127:1353-1360.

2 Genzyme Corporation. Aubagio (teriflunomide) prescribing information (2012). Revised October 2014a. http://products.sanofi.us/aubagio/aubagio.pdf. Accessed April 6, 2016.

3 Langer-Gould A, Huang SM, Gupta R, et al. Exclusive breastfeeding and the risk of postpartum relapses in women with multiple sclerosis. *Arch Neurol*. 66:958-963.

4 Pakpoor J, Disanto G, Lacey MV, Hellwig K, Giovannoni G, Ramagopalan SV. Breastfeeding and multiple sclerosis relapses: a meta-analysis. *J Neurol*. 2012;259:2246-2248.

5 Airas L, Jalkanen A, Alanen A, Pirttilä T, Marttila RJ. Breast-feeding, postpartum and prepregnancy disease activity in multiple sclerosis. *Neurology*. 2010; 75:474-476.

6 Confavreux C, Hutchinson M, Hours MM, Cortinovis-Tourniaire P, Moreau T. Rate of pregnancy-related relapse in multiple sclerosis. Pregnancy in Multiple Sclerosis Group. *N Engl J Med*. 1998;339:285-291.

7 Houtchens MK, Kolb CM. Multiple sclerosis and pregnancy: therapeutic considerations. *J. Neurol*. 2013;260:1202-1214.

8 Cree BAC. Update on reproductive safety of current and emerging disease-modifying therapies for multiple sclerosis. *Mult. Scler*. 2013;19:835-843.

9 Achiron A, Kishner I, Dolev M, et al. Effect of intravenous immunoglobulin treatment on pregnancy and postpartum-related relapses in multiple sclerosis. *J Neurol*. 2004;251:1133-1137.

10 Haas J. High dose IVIG in the postpartum period for prevention of exacerbations in MS. *Mult Scler*. 2000;6(suppl 2):S18-20; Disc S33.

11 Fragoso YD, Adoni T, Alves-Leon SV, et al. Postpartum treatment with immunoglobulin does not prevent relapses of multiple sclerosis in the mother. *Health Care Women Int*. 2014;1-9.

Other Multiple
Sclerosis-Related Disorders

Neuromyelitis optica

Elias Sotirchos and Shiv Saidha

History

A 45-year-old woman with a history of right-sided optic neuritis (ON) with severe residual vision loss presented with rapidly evolving bilateral lower extremity weakness. She reported that approximately 7 days prior to presentation, she noticed a band-like 'squeezing' sensation across her chest. Over the next few days, she developed progressively worsening weakness and numbness in both lower extremities, culminating in an inability to ambulate. Furthermore, she experienced significant urinary urgency and frequency, constipation, and had episodes of urinary and bowel incontinence.

Examination

Her neurologic exam was notable for the following: a right relative afferent pupillary defect, right optic disc pallor, and 20/200 visual acuity in the right eye. She also had bilateral lower extremity weakness (range from 2/5 to 3/5 strength, flexors affected more severely than extensors – consistent with a pyramidal pattern of weakness), as well as hyperreflexia in both lower extremities, extensor plantar responses bilaterally, and a sensory level to pinprick, light touch, and vibration at approximately T4.

Investigations

A brain MRI was unremarkable and an MRI of the spinal cord demonstrated a large T2 hyperintense lesion within the spinal cord extending from T1–T9

© Springer International Publishing Switzerland 2017   139
P.S. Giacomini (ed.), *Case Studies in Multiple Sclerosis*,
DOI 10.1007/978-3-319-31190-6_19

that exhibited patchy enhancement from T2–T7 following the administration of gadolinium on T1-weighted sequences (Figure 19.1). Spinal fluid analyses revealed 67 white blood cells (WBC)/mm^3 (70% mononuclear, 30% polymorphonuclear), normal protein and glucose, and negative oligoclonal bands.

Routine laboratory studies were unremarkable and HIV, syphilis, antinuclear antibody, collapsin-response mediator protein 5 antibody, anti-Ro/La antibodies, erythrocyte sedimentation rate, and C-reactive protein were all normal or negative. Testing for serum autoantibodies targeting aquaporin-4 (AQP4) was positive.

Outcome

The patient was diagnosed with neuromyelitis optica (NMO). She was treated with a 5-day course of high-dose intravenous steroids (methylprednisolone 1 g daily), followed by an oral prednisone taper. She had minimal improvement and an intravascular catheter was placed and plasma exchange initiated. After completion of five sessions of plasma

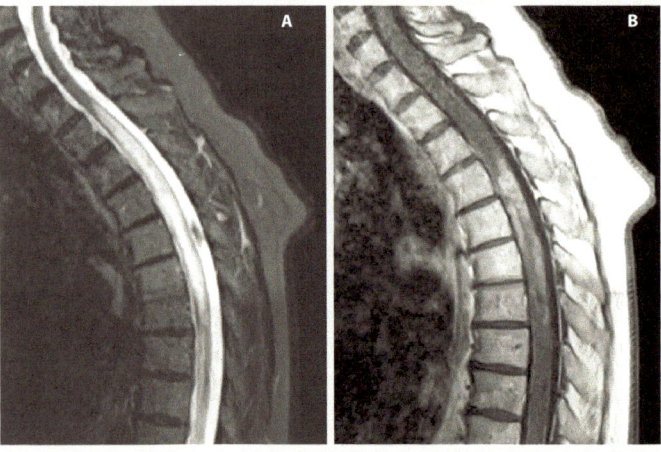

Figure 19.1 Sagittal T2-weighted sequence (A) showing a longitudinally extensive spinal cord lesion extending from T1–T9. Sagittal T1-weighted sequence (**B**) obtained after gadolinium administration demonstrates heterogeneous enhancement extending from T2–T7 within the core of the lesion demonstrated in Panel A.

exchange performed on alternate days, she exhibited significant improvement. Thereafter, she was commenced on treatment with rituximab in order to reduce the risk for future relapses.

Discussion

This case illustrates a typical NMO presentation, also known as Devic's disease. As the name implies, NMO is an inflammatory disorder of the central nervous system, with a predilection to afflict the spinal cord and optic nerves. NMO is a distinct disorder from multiple sclerosis (MS) and has been associated with the presence of autoantibodies (eg, NMO-immunglobulin G [IgG]) directed against the water channel AQP-4, a finding that is present in roughly 75% of patients with NMO [1,2]. NMO-IgG seropositivity is regarded as highly specific and supportive for the diagnosis of NMO [2]. The differences in demographics, epidemiology, clinical presentation, course, imaging, and laboratory findings between NMO and MS are outlined in Table 19.1.

In the vast majority of patients with NMO, the disease follows a relapsing course with bouts of ON and/or transverse myelitis (TM), which usually occur separately but may also occur simultaneously, a presentation which should raise a high suspicion for the diagnosis of NMO [3].

Optic neuritis

ON is characterized by acute onset visual loss which develops over a period of hours to days, frequently associated with eye pain that is exacerbated by eye movements. Findings on clinical examination include decreased visual acuity, abnormal color vision, a relative afferent pupillary defect which is usually present in ON provided that the contralateral eye and optic nerve are healthy, various patterns of visual field defects (including central scotomas, diffuse vision loss, arcuate, hemianopic, altitudinal and cecocentral defects) and optic disc edema, which may be seen in about one-third of patients with ON [4]. Certain clinical characteristics are suggestive of NMO-associated ON, including increased severity with worse visual outcomes, often resulting in blindness, chiasmal involvement which may cause bitemporal hemianopia, and altitudinal visual field defects (which is also a characteristic of ischemic optic neuropathy) [5,6].

	Multiple sclerosis (MS)	Neuromyelitis optica (NMO)
Age of onset (median)	29	39
Sex ratio (female:male)	2:1	6:1 to 9:1
Prevalence	~100 per 100,000 population in North America and Europe	0.5–4 per 100,000 population
Initial clinical course	90% relapsing-remitting 10% primary progressive	80–90% relapsing-remitting 10–20% monophasic
Secondary progressive course	Frequent	Rare
Relapse severity and recovery	Variable but often good recovery from individual relapses	Often severe with poor recovery

Brain MRI findings	• Periventricular white matter, ovoid-shaped lesions perpendicular to ventricles reflecting perivenular distribution
	• Juxtacortical white matter
	• Corpus callosum
	• Infratentorial
	• Cortical lesions (not routinely visualized with conventional MRI)
		• Usually normal or non-specific white matter lesions
		• Characteristic lesions involve the periependymal surfaces of the ventricular system
		  – Lateral ventricles: periventricular adjacent to ependymal lining; ependymal surface of corpus callosum
		  – 3rd ventricle and cerebral aqueduct: lesions of the diencephalon (eg, hypothalamus, thalamus)
		  – 4th ventricle: area postrema and other areas of the brainstem; cerbellum
		• 10% of patients with NMO will have lesions on MRI that appear to be consistent with MS

Optic nerve MRI findings	• Short lesions usually affecting the anterior segments of the optic nerves	• Longer lesions and posterior/optic chiasm involvement • Often bilateral involvement
Spinal cord MRI findings	• Short-segment lesions (1–2 vertebral segments) • Asymmetric, peripheral lesions involving the white matter tracts causing partial spinal cord syndromes	• Frequently longitudinally extensive (≥3 vertebral segments) • Large central lesions involving gray and white matter causing complete spinal cord syndromes

Table 19.1 Comparison of demographics, epidemiology, clinical presentation, course, MRI, CSF findings and treatment between multiple sclerosis and neuromyelitis optica (continues on next page).

	Multiple sclerosis (MS)	Neuromyelitis optica (NMO)
CSF cell count/ differential (during relapses)	Usually mild mononuclear pleiocytosis (<50/mm³)	Often prominent pleiocytosis (>50mm³ in ~35% of patients) with mononuclear and polymorphonuclear cells present
CSF oligoclonal bands	~85%	15–30%
Treatment of relapses	• Glucocorticoids • Plasma exchange (if severe and poor response to glucocorticoids)	• Glucocorticoids • Plasma exchange required more frequently than in MS given increased attack severity
Common treatments for relapse prevention	• Interferon beta-1a and -1b • Glatiramer acetate • Natalizumab • Fingolimod • Dimethyl fumarate • Teriflunomide • Alemtuzumab	• Rituximab • Mycophenolate mofetil • Prednisone • Methotrexate • Azathioprine

Table 19.1 Comparison of demographics, epidemiology, clinical presentation, course, MRI, CSF findings and treatment between multiple sclerosis and neuromyelitis optica (continued). CSF, cerebrospinal fluid;.

Additionally, while NMO-associated ON is often unilateral, simultaneous bilateral ON or rapid sequential ON may occur not infrequently and this has been shown to account for 11–20% of initial presentations of NMO [5]. By contrast, simultaneous bilateral ON is rare in adult MS and, consequently, this should raise suspicion for NMO.

MRI in NMO-associated ON may show thickening of the sheath of the optic nerve, T2 hyperintensities in the optic nerve, and post-contrast enhancement on T1-weighted sequences, findings that may be seen in MS-associated ON as well [7]. However, longitudinally extensive lesions (involving greater than half the length of the optic nerve from the orbit to the chiasm), more posterior involvement of the optic nerve, and/or chiasmal involvement have been shown to be characteristics associated with NMO.

Transverse myelitis

TM typically presents with limb weakness, with the extent of involvement depending on the level and laterality of the lesion, sensory loss (below the level of the lesion), and bladder, bowel, and/or sexual dysfunction.

Often patients with TM will complain of a band-like sensation at the level of the lesion that may develop initially, before the onset of other symptoms. The onset of TM symptoms is usually over several hours to days; hyperacute presentations with symptoms reaching nadir within 4 hours should raise the possibility of alternative etiologies and, in particular, vascular myelopathies [8].

NMO-related TM is typically characterized by a preferential involvement of the central gray matter of the spinal cord, which often results in symmetric limb weakness [7]. This may be visualized on MRI axial sections of the spinal cord. However, the hallmark manifestation of NMO is longitudinally extensive TM, which is defined as a contiguous lesion that spans ≥3 vertebral segments [3,7]. By contrast, MS-associated TM is frequently asymmetric, involves the white matter, and is characterized by short segment lesions that are usually less than two vertebral segments in length [3]. During the acute phase of TM, enhancement is seen on post-gadolinium T1-weighted sequences, indicating active inflammation and breakdown of the blood–brain barrier. Spinal cord enlargement may also be seen during active inflammation due to edema-related swelling.

Other clinical syndromes

Other clinical syndromes may also occur in NMO, either in isolation or in addition to more classical involvement of the optic nerves and spinal cord. A characteristic location of NMO brainstem lesions is adjacent to the fourth ventricle in the dorsal brainstem. NMO affliction of the area postrema in the dorsal medulla results in a syndrome that manifests with intractable hiccups, nausea, and vomiting [6,7]. Lesions in this location may be contiguous with cervical spinal cord lesions. Furthermore, diencephalic lesions surrounding the third ventricle and cerebral aqueduct may also be observed in NMO [6,7]. Such lesions may result in hypothalamic dysfunction with diverse clinical manifestation including narcolepsy, autonomic dysfunction, endocrine abnormalities, and behavioral changes.

Brain MRI

A brain MRI in NMO is classically described as being either normal or demonstrating non-specific white matter abnormalities. However, it is now recognized that brain MRI abnormalities may actually be seen in up to as many as 85% of patients with NMO [7]. Characteristic locations of NMO brain lesions include the periependymal surfaces surrounding the ventricular system (especially the dorsal medulla and diencephalon), the corpus callosum (diffuse lesions), and the corticospinal tracts, often contiguously involving the internal capsule and cerebral peduncle. Other rarer presentations are associated with the presence of large, confluent, tumefactive lesions involving the subcortical or deep white matter. Additionally, it should be noted that as many as 16% of patients with NMO fulfill the MRI criteria for an MS diagnosis [6].

Laboratory findings

The laboratory hallmark of NMO is the presence of NMO-IgG, a serum autoantibody that is directed against AQP4 and that is thought to be intimately involved in the pathogenesis of the disorder. This finding is highly specific for NMO; however, sensitivity in patients with a clinical diagnosis of NMO is approximately 75% [2].

Cerebrospinal fluid (CSF) analysis during relapses often reveals pleiocytosis, which in as many as 35% of patients may be greater than 50 WBC/mm^3 with a typically mononuclear predominance, although neutrophils and/or eosinophils may also be present [9]. In MS, the CSF WBC count is typically less than 50 WBC/mm^3 and is usually exclusively mononuclear, so these features may also help in differentiating NMO from MS. Additionally, CSF-specific oligoclonal bands are present in approximately 85% of patients with MS, indicating intrathecal antibody synthesis, while in NMO, they are less commonly detected (approximately 15–30% of patients) [9].

Of note, NMO is strongly associated with other systemic autoimmune diseases such as autoimmune thyroiditis, systemic lupus erythematosus, and Sjögren's syndrome, among others [10]. Testing for autoantibodies associated with these autoimmune conditions in patients with NMO, even in the absence of clinical manifestations, demonstrates that a significant proportion of patients with NMO harbor additional autoantibodies (eg, up to 43% of patients with NMO are seropositive for antinuclear antibodies).

Diagnosis

The initial diagnostic criteria for NMO were published by Wingerchuk et al in 2006 [11] and required the following:

- optic neuritis;
- acute myelitis; and
- at least two of three supportive criteria:
  - contiguous spinal cord MRI lesion extending ≥3 vertebral segments,
  - brain MRI not meeting diagnostic criteria for MS, and/or
  - NMO-IgG seropositivity.

However, the widespread introduction of NMO-IgG testing has since identified patients that are NMO-IgG seropositive but that do not fulfill the 2006 criteria for the diagnosis of NMO; this includes patients with isolated ON, TM, or brain lesions typical of NMO as described previously (eg, brainstem or diencephalic lesions). These syndromes were subsequently encompassed by the umbrella term 'NMO spectrum disorders' (NMOSD) and have been linked to an increased risk of future relapse; therefore, it is recommended that the approach to their treatment does not differ from that of NMO.

It is worth noting that revised diagnostic criteria for NMO have recently been proposed [6]. These revised diagnostic guidelines utilize the term NMOSD as a unifying modified term that covers both conventional NMO, as well as NMOSD as conceptualized in a more traditional sense. The revised diagnostic criteria stratify NMSOD according to NMO-IgG seropositivity status. In patients that are NMO-IgG seropositive, making a diagnosis of NMO is now somewhat easier and less stringent. The criteria allow NMOSD diagnosis in NMO-IgG seropositive patients with the occurrence of at least one of six core clinical characteristics including affliction of the following regions: optic nerve, spinal cord, area postrema of the dorsal medulla, brainstem, diencephalon, or cerebrum. In patients that are NMO-IgG seronegative, making a diagnosis of NMO is more stringent. Such patients must experience two or more different core clinical characteristics and exhibit other supportive MRI characteristics in order to enhance diagnostic specificity. At least one of the clinical events must be one of the three most common clinical characteristics of NMOSD: ON, TM (additional requirement: longitudinally extensive myelitis MRI lesion), or an area postrema clinical syndrome (additional requirement: associated medullary MRI lesion). The two required core characteristics may occur within a single clinical attack or over the course of multiple attacks.

Treatment

The mainstay of treatment of relapses in NMO is intravenous high-dose glucocorticoids administered for 3–5 days [12,13]. For patients with severe relapses or who do not respond to glucocorticoids alone, plasma exchange is indicated [12–14]. Because NMO is a relapsing-remitting inflammatory disorder, long-term immunosuppression is warranted in order to prevent future relapses. The most frequently utilized medications for this purpose include mycophenolate mofetil, rituximab, azathioprine, and methotrexate [12,13]. An important point regarding the treatment of NMO is that the treatments utilized in MS for prevention of relapses are not effective in NMO, and some MS disease-modifying therapies (eg, interferon, natalizumab, and fingolimod) may actually cause exacerbations of NMO [13]. This further emphasizes the importance of differentiating NMO from MS and early, accurate diagnosis.

Clinical pearls

- NMO is an inflammatory disorder of the central nervous system that predominantly affects the spinal cord and optic nerves (eg, TM, ON).
- ON in NMO may be bilateral or rapidly sequential, cause severe vision loss, and affect the posterior regions of the optic nerve and chiasm.
- TM in NMO causes large central lesions, causing complete spinal cord syndromes.
- Spinal cord lesions in NMO are frequently longitudinally extensive (spanning ≥3 vertebral segments).
- The brainstem may be involved in NMO, especially the dorsal medulla including the area postrema, causing a syndrome manifesting with intractable hiccups, nausea, and vomiting.

- The hypothalamus may be involved in NMO causing hypothalamic dysfunction with presenting symptoms including narcolepsy, autonomic dysfunction, endocrine abnormalities, and behavioral changes.
- NMO is associated with seropositivity of anti-AQP4 IgG antibodies (NMO-IgG) in approximately 75% of patients.
- NMO is strongly associated with systemic autoimmune diseases including autoimmune thyroiditis, systemic lupus erythematosus, and Sjögren's syndrome.
- Relapses in NMO are treated with intravenous glucocorticoids and plasma exchange (if severe or no response to steroids).
- Long-term immunotherapy is warranted in NMO to prevent relapses and includes mycophenolate mofetil, rituximab, azathioprine, or methotrexate.
- Treatments used to prevent relapses in MS are not effective in NMO and in some instances may cause exacerbations of NMO.

References

1   Lennon VA, Kryzer TJ, Pittock SJ, Verkman AS, Hinson SR. IgG marker of optic-spinal multiple sclerosis binds to the aquaporin-4 water channel. *J Exp Med*. 2005;202:473-477.
2   Jarius S, Wildemann B. Aquaporin-4 antibodies (NMO-IgG) as a serological marker of neuromyelitis optica: a critical review of the literature. *Brain Pathol*. 2013;23:661-683.
3   Wingerchuk DM, Lennon VA, Lucchinetti CF, Pittock SJ, Weinshenker BG. The spectrum of neuromyelitis optica. *Lancet Neurol*. 2007;6:805-815.
4   The clinical profile of optic neuritis. Experience of the Optic Neuritis Treatment Trial. Optic Neuritis Study Group. *Arch Ophthal*. 1991;109:1673-1678.
5   Levin MH, Bennett JL, Verkman AS. Optic neuritis in neuromyelitis optica. *Prog Retin Eye Res*. 2013;36:159-171.
6   Wingerchuk DM, Banwell B, Bennett JL, et al. International consensus diagnostic criteria for neuromyelitis optica spectrum disorders. *Neurology*. 2015;85:177-189.
7   Kim HJ, Paul F, Lana-Peixoto MA, et al. MRI characteristics of neuromyelitis optica spectrum disorder: an international update. *Neurology*. 2015;84:1165-1173.
8   Transverse Myelitis Consortium Working Group. Proposed diagnostic criteria and nosology of acute transverse myelitis. *Neurology*. 2002;59:499-505.
9   Morrow MJ, Wingerchuk D. Neuromyelitis optica. *J Neuroophthalmol*.2012;32:154-166.
10 Wingerchuk DM, Weinshenker BG. The emerging relationship between neuromyelitis optica and systemic rheumatologic autoimmune disease. *Mult Scler*. 2012;18:5-10.
11 Wingerchuk DM, Lennon VA, Pittock SJ, Lucchinetti CF, Weinshenker BG. Revised diagnostic criteria for neuromyelitis optica. *Neurology*. 2006;66:1485-1489.
12 Kimbrough DJ, Fujihara K, Jacob A, et al. Treatment of neuromyelitis optica: review and recommendations. *Mult Scler Relat Disord*. 2012;1:180-187.
13 Papadopoulos MC, Bennett JL, Verkman AS. Treatment of neuromyelitis optica: state-of-the-art and emerging therapies. *Nature Rev Neurol*. 2014;10:493-506.

14   Abboud H, Petrak A, Mealy M, Sasidharan S, Siddique L, Levy M. Treatment of acute relapses in neuromyelitis optica: steroids alone versus steroids plus plasma exchange. *Multiple Scler.* 2016;22:185-192.